C000100022

PRAISE FOR
MY LIFE IN STITCHES

"*My Life in Stitches* provides the reader with a practical and heart-warming guide to dealing with a chronic heart diagnosis and transplant. This book is a must-read for patients, families, and medical teams dealing with long-term illness, surgery, and recovery."

—ROLAND MONTEMAYOR, M.A., MARRIAGE
AND FAMILY COUNSELOR

"As an advanced practice nurse who specializes in critical care, I believe patients and their loved ones, as well as healthcare professionals, will benefit from reading this humorous tale of life and death. There are so few resources available to recommend to patients who are experiencing life-threatening illness, and I am pleased to be able to share this book."

—REBECCA LONG, MS, RN, CNS, FORMER
CHAIR OF THE AMERICAN ASSOCIATION OF
CRITICAL CARE NURSES CERTIFICATION
BOARD

"An amazing element in Darla's story is a prevailing sense of humor that allows her to get beyond her personal pain and find a funny moment — even at her own expense. Whether she is calling herself a P.T. Barnum sideshow freak at a medical meeting or an LVAD Barbie among fellow patients, Darla's heroic struggle is both an inspiration and proof that the will to live is the greatest medicine of all."

—ANNA WILCOXSON, AUTHOR OF THE
SECRETS AND PROMISES SERIES

My Life
in
STITCHES

A HEART TRANSPLANT
SURVIVOR STORY

DARLA A. CALVET, PHD

FROM THE TINY ACORN...
GROWS THE MIGHTY OAK

This book is a memoir. It reflects the author's present recollections of experiences over time. Some names and characteristics have been changed, some events have been compressed, and some dialogue has been recreated. The author in no way represents any company, corporation, or brand mentioned herein.

My Life in Stitches
Copyright © 2023 Darla A. Calvet. All rights reserved.

Printed in the United States of America. For information, address
Acorn Publishing, LLC
3943 Irvine Blvd. Ste. 218, Irvine, CA 92602

www.acornpublishingllc.com

Interior design by Kat Ross
Cover design by Damonza

Anti-Piracy Warning: The unauthorized reproduction or distribution of a copyrighted work is illegal. Criminal copyright infringement, including infringement without monetary gain, is investigated by the FBI and is punishable by up to five years in federal prison and a fine of $250,000.

All rights reserved. No part of this book may be used or reproduced in any manner whatsoever, including Internet usage, without written permission from the author.

ISBN-13: 979-8-88528-056-3 (hardcover)
ISBN-13: 979-8-88528-055-6 (paperback)
Library of Congress Control Number: 2023903653

This book is lovingly dedicated to my donor Alex, his family, and my tribe who got me through transplant. Specifically, my husband Patrick Calvet, daughters Claire and Annie Calvet, and our friends and family. I would not be here without your love and support.

THE PRIEST AND THE PEANUT BUTTER SANDWICH

THE FIRST TIME I heard the word "transplant," I was lying in a grimy hospital bed in the urgent care unit, surrounded by flimsy plastic curtains with 1960s daisies on them. A pudgy nurse with bleached-blonde hair and stained tie-dyed scrubs came in to take my blood pressure. "Do you know anyone who can get you on the transplant list?" she asked. I looked at her in disbelief, mumbling, "Oh my God, am I that sick?!" I had been feeling run-down in the past month or so but had no idea that my condition was life-threatening. She stuck a thermometer under my tongue and said, "Well, your heart is not pumping very well, and it would help if you knew someone who could get you on one of those transplant waiting lists." She pulled the flimsy curtain tight and left the room. I blinked back tears in a state of shock. My journey to transplant had begun.

Shortly after the nurse left, my parents entered my room. They looked frightened and sleep-deprived, with dark grey rings around their eyes, resembling human racoons. My mom and dad had very different personalities, and their responses to my newly diagnosed illness were just as varied. My dad, a survivor of open-heart surgery, was supportive and empathetic. After hearing my diagnosis, he put his meaty hand on my arm and said compassionately, "I'm sorry you're sick, honey." My mom, a feisty Italian woman, was less sympathetic. She snapped, "Well, I am not surprised that you're sick. You in graduate school working full time and have two little kids."

As much as her words stung, she was right. Like many working moms in the early 2000s, I was clearly overdoing it. Now, my body was paying the price. I was a college administrator at a local university in San Diego. I was also enrolled in a doctoral program in Higher Education with a goal of finishing in four years while working full-time. I had two young daughters. Claire was ten years old and in fourth grade; Annie was seven years old and in first grade. There was far too much on my plate, and I was in denial about my overcommitment. Now, as I lay in the hospital bed, I began to realize that the ongoing stress had done permanent damage to my body. I felt horrible mentally and physically.

One of the admitting doctors thought that I might have caught a respiratory infection caused by a virus. It was 2003, and a mystery virus called "SARS" had come over to the United States from China. My doctor theorized that perhaps the virus had "jumped" from my lung tissue to my heart tissue in an aggressive manner, causing heart failure. This was only an educated guess. The final diagnosis given to me by the admitting physician was "idiopathic dilated cardiomyopathy." In layman's terms, this meant a diagnosis of congestive heart failure (CHF) by an unknown cause. I had to face the reality that being an overworked wife, mom, and career woman was not manageable. The fight to reclaim my life and body had begun.

The night before my admission to the emergency room, I had felt queasy and sick to my stomach. I sluggishly crawled into bed around 10:00 p.m. after returning from an exhausting business trip to our university's headquarters in San Francisco and had barely completed the trip home. I attended a late lunch work meeting in Union Square and felt nauseous as soon as I got up to leave the table. I walked to Union Street for a taxi to the airport and promptly regurgitated my salad on the sidewalk in front of a bunch of horrified Japanese tourists. I rarely had stomach issues and assumed that I had food poisoning. Embarrassed, I snuck into a local Starbucks bathroom and changed my clothes before boarding the flight home.

The next morning, I woke up with swollen ankles the size of grapefruits. This medical condition is called "cardiac edema." It results from an overworked heart that is no longer able to pump fluids such as blood and water around the body. This results in pools of fluid in the patient's stomach, ankles, feet, legs, arms, hands, and other areas. As I looked down at my swollen ankles, I started to panic. Something was seriously wrong, and I could no longer deny how tired and worn out I had been for the last year. I had gone in for a full physical the week before the trip, complaining of being unable to breathe. My doctor gave me a clean bill of health and told me I had asthma. The medication he prescribed could have killed me. I would later learn that over 96 percent of females with heart disease are misdiagnosed every year by doctors, which may explain why it is the number one killer of all women in the United States.

My husband Pat is not known to mince words. Seeing my grapefruit-sized ankles, he blurted, "What's that?!" to no one in particular.

I quietly responded, "I don't know, but something is horribly wrong."

In a panic, we called Pat's sister, Helene, who is an infectious disease doctor, for advice. She listened to my symptoms and replied, "Go to the closest emergency room. Now. Do it! I will drive down in an hour to help you." We hurried our girls into our family van, then drove off to the hospital. The girls fell back to sleep, and we rode to the emergency room in silence. An overwhelming sense of dread hung over us. The five-minute drive to the ER felt like an hour.

My fears that something was seriously wrong were confirmed as we checked into the musty, overcrowded emergency room. I showed the admitting clerk my elephantine ankles, and she immediately bumped me to the head of the line. I was out of breath and wheezed repeatedly. I thanked her on my way to the exam room and gasped, "I can't breathe."

She looked me straight in the eye and responded, "You have a heart virus. I can already tell." She was correct in her diagnosis.

After being quickly assessed in the triage area, the silver-haired, haggard-looking physician on duty looked at my vital signs and ankles. He frowned. "It looks like you are in heart failure. They are going to transport you to the regular hospital for tests and admittance." Before I could plead with him for more information, he was gone. I noticed that the man in the bed next to me began urinating in a bedpan. I wanted to scream but shut my eyes instead. I prayed to God that this was some kind of horrible dream, and I would wake up in my normal life. I was only thirty-nine years old.

A half hour passed, and two young male paramedics loaded me up on a sitting gurney. It was bright yellow and black and reminded me of a giant bumblebee robot transformer. Although I must have looked monstrous with my slicked-back hair and sweating forehead, they were kind to me and tried to be reassuring.

"Okay miss, we will be transporting you over to the main hospital now," said one of them as he lifted up the giant gurney.

The half-mile trip between the emergency room and the main hospital was a ridiculous exercise in logistics. It took them twenty minutes to get me loaded and buckled in, then five minutes to drive over to the main building and another twenty to unload me. They placed me in a temporary patient holding room on the main floor of the hospital, where I encountered the pudgy peroxided nurse.

My husband Pat had gone home to leave the kids with some trusted neighbors while I waited for more treatment. I sat alone in the holding room in a despondent state. After hours of sitting alone considering my bleak diagnosis, a tall, older priest with a shock of white hair entered the room, smiling. I took one look at him and whispered, "Oh my God. Are you here to administer the Last Rites?"

In a predictable Irish brogue, he took my hand and replied, "No, child. I am just here to see if you are hungry. I know you have been here a while. I brought you a bit of something."

He pulled his hand from his shirt pocket and produced a tiny peanut butter sandwich, neatly wrapped in plastic. I had been at the hospital for over eighteen hours and had been given nothing but water and intravenous fluid. "Oh, thank you, Father," I said with relief. "Yes, I am a bit hungry, and I would love that." We both shared a good laugh before he gave me a standard blessing and continued his rounds. I was going to need it.

The first lesson I learned as a heart transplant patient is that a sense of humor is vital on the road to recovery. You cannot survive without it.

2

THE FIRST ATTENDING CARDIOLOGIST

AFTER LYING in the makeshift hospital room for five more hours, the on-call hospital cardiologist finally arrived. He was a middle-aged, handsome Indian man in an expensive Armani double-breasted suit with diamond rings on both hands. As he bent over my bed to take my vitals, those manicured doctor hands projected a lovely prism of rainbow light across the dark, gloomy hospital room. I watched the rainbow orbs dance across the ceiling as he began his examination of me. It's funny the things you notice when you are confined to a hospital bed with nowhere to go.

He removed a stethoscope from his breast pocket and listened to my chest, intently. After a moment or two, he clucked sympathetically and took my sweaty hand in his. He averted eye contact, staring at the wall behind me. He sighed deeply, saying, "Carla, I have some bad news for you. You have idiopathic dilated cardiomyopathy." It did not rattle me that this attending cardiologist had called me by the wrong name as he delivered this serious diagnosis. My mom named me after the only female Little Rascal, "Darla." She loved her precociousness and the spunky attitude she had with the other boy Rascals. I was used to people mistakenly calling me Carla at this point in my life. What did upset me was the scary-sounding diagnosis.

When I pressed this doctor to explain idiopathic dilated cardiomyopathy to me, he glanced down at his Rolex watch and said, "We will need time to figure out what is going on here. I will have you discharged to rest at home and then see you in my office in two weeks." The vague, glassy words hung awkwardly in the air above us. The undercurrent to his response was, *I am not going to tell you anything else at this point in time, so there is no use trying to learn more.* I would learn that this type of generalized information is often given by physicians when they do not want to commit to a more defined diagnosis without conducting tests. In our lawsuit-ridden society, I cannot blame them for trying to protect themselves.

The attending cardiologist continued to speak in a hushed, hurried tone, as if he wanted to get home to his family for dinner. "I am very sorry that you are so young to have this condition. You are only thirty-nine years old. This is a very early age to have this illness."

Somehow, though his words were meant to comfort me, they had the opposite effect. My self-blaming was kicking into full gear. I had internal racing thoughts such as, "I should have lost that baby weight," and "If only I hadn't worked so much since becoming a mom." This thinking is common among newly diagnosed patients. The doctors do not have to scold us; we do it to ourselves.

I was extremely anxious and wanted answers on my condition immediately, not within the next month. I would soon realize that being a cardiology patient includes an ample amount of waiting time and patience, which most "type A" cardiology patients lack. As a cardiac patient, you are expected to promptly undergo tests when requested, then wait for lengthy periods until those results are available. The attending cardiologist had not run another echocardiogram since I had been admitted to the hospital. When I asked him why we could not do more tests, he simply replied, "It can wait." I decided that if he would not provide me with the answers I needed, I would find another cardiologist who would.

The next lesson I learned as a heart transplant patient is that time is of the essence when fighting heart disease, and you must be your own advocate for getting the highest quality care available.

3

DR. HELENE

AFTER MORE THAN TWENTY-FOUR HOURS, I was discharged from the local hospital by the attending physician and returned home. I had left our home like any other normal mom, happy in my suburban world. Now I was returning home in my new role as a chronically ill patient who would be battling for her life. In my former life, I thought twice before even taking aspirin. In my new life as a CHF patient, I would be enduring drugs, devices, and all types of rigorous tests in the quest for information on my condition. On this road to recovery, I was going to lean harder on my family and closest friends more than I had ever imagined.

The first member of our recovery team was waiting for us at home. Dr. Helene, my husband's younger sister, was a top-notch infectious disease doctor who had finished UCLA medical school at the tender age of twenty-eight. The most endearing thing about Dr. Helene was that she still cared about people after becoming a physician. She had driven down from Orange County to San Diego to help us as soon as my husband Pat called her to inquire about my grapefruit-sized ankles.

While Pat and I were dealing with life at the hospital, Dr. Helene had taken control of our domestic situation. She comforted our daughters, grocery shopped, and had dinner waiting for us on the table when we arrived home. Pat and I were exhausted from the ordeal of the last twenty-four hours and were grateful for her help. Ever the optimist, Dr. Helene greeted us at the door, smiling. She quipped, "You know, guys, there are easier ways to take a vacation."

We sat down to a "heart healthy" dinner of low sodium tomato soup and grilled chicken breasts. Over dinner, Dr. Helene became a bit more serious and began to instruct us on what to do next after my hospital discharge. "I called your physician at the hospital and spoke with him, although it was hard to understand his Indian accent. He told me that you needed to be on a cardiac low-sodium diet of no more than twelve hundred milligrams of sodium per day."

I jokingly replied, "Helene, I could swallow that much salt swimming across La Jolla Cove." While we all laughed, I knew that my love of the saltshaker was going to have to go away for quite a while. Maybe even forever. The tasteless tomato soup and rubbery chicken breasts on the plate in front of me were hardly what I would call "comfort food." This was all part of my "new normal" after my CHF diagnosis and I was not quite liking it.

Once we put our two daughters to bed, I sat down with Dr. Helene over some tea (caffeine-free, of course). I looked her in the eyes and said, "Alright, do not sugar-coat this for me. What is CHF and why did the nurse say I needed a transplant?"

In her best matter-of-fact consulting physician tone, Dr. Helene replied, "Honestly, I do not know. My guess is that your heart somehow became enlarged, and it can no longer pump blood through your body the way it should. This is what caused the cardiac edema in your feet. They will need to do more tests. I am not a cardiologist, so I cannot really speculate on this. What I can tell you is that you need to rest, eat low sodium meals, and get the tests your doctor asks you to take."

This was not what I wanted to hear. Dr. Helene had been a saint, and I realized that I should not be angry with her for not knowing what was going on. I leaned in closer toward her and took her hand, whispering, "Am I going to die? Is it really true I will need a transplant? What if I don't survive?" The panic in my voice was escalating with each question. Within a mere day, I had gone from a healthy mom and wife to a very sick person who wanted answers that no one could provide. As I assumed this new sick role, I had never felt lonelier or more scared in my life.

Dr. Helene gave me a hug. "It's really in God's hands."

I returned her embrace and went to the bedroom for my first of many good cries.

The next morning, Dr. Helene was up early packing her electric car. She had a very busy work schedule as a public health physician at the Long Beach California Department of Health and Human Services. We made small talk as she prepared to drive away, thanking her for her time and support. While she smiled and kept the conversation light, I could tell from her brittle posture and frightened eyes that we were in for a hell of a journey. In the months and years to come, Dr. Helene would become one of our greatest advocates in the fight to save my failing health. She was the best sister-in-law I could have hoped for, and a world-class physician and patient advocate.

My fondest memory of Dr. Helene throughout this entire process was a funny one. On Thanksgiving Day in 2014, I was forced to stay at the hospital after the team had told me I might be able to go home. I was highly disappointed and missed my family terribly. To buoy my spirits, Dr. Helene came to visit me. She walked in with her white lab coat and stethoscope, with a turkey hat perched on her head. She made me laugh and brought a smile to my very grumpy face. These are the kind of people one needs around during the road to transplant.

The next lesson I learned as a heart transplant patient is to accept help from those who offer it, especially medical professionals. They will become vital members of your treatment support team.

4

IF A TREE FALLS IN THE FOREST

DESPITE THE FACT that thousands of people get transplanted every year, the journey can be a lonely one. The transplant patient often spends many hours in solitude each day while friends and loved ones go on with their normal work and home lives. To help ease this sense of loneliness, the day after I returned home I drove to the closest bookstore looking for reference books on heart conditions, CHF, and transplant. As I wandered through the health section, I saw entire walls of books dedicated to cancer, diabetes, and mental health, but not a single book on heart disease, transplant, or recovery. This blew my mind. Heart disease is the number one killer of men and women in America. I had to be looking in the wrong section.

After searching fruitlessly on my own for thirty minutes, I found a nerdy-looking millennial wearing a bookstore nametag on her employee lanyard. "Hi Dakota, do you think you could help me find a book on heart disease?" I asked. She gave me a blank stare and replied, "Um, let me get you my manager." Cardiac illness is unfamiliar to most people under thirty unless they have dealt with someone in their family having it. Fifteen minutes later, a white-haired male manager with coke-bottle glasses shuffled out from the stockroom. "What is it you want, miss? Something about heart surgery?"

Not wanting to share any personal details, I tried to keep my conversation brief. "Well, I am doing some research on heart problems and could not find any books on it in your medical or self-help sections. Do you know why that is?"

He thought for a moment, then said, "Well, heart disease is pretty depressing. Most people do not want to read about it. Come to think of it, a few people have come in here looking for the same type of help, but we do not have anything except books on being a caregiver."

I wondered why there were no patient books written on heart disease, which kills so many Americans every day. Disappointed, I bought myself a copy of *Vanity Fair* and a Godiva dark chocolate almond bar, then headed home. The American Heart Association offered some helpful information, but not much from the patient perspective. How could this be? People had been dying from heart disease for decades, *yet no one was talking about it.*

Once I returned home, I began searching on Amazon for some type of heart disease survival story or inspirational book. Instead, I found books like *Grey's Anatomy for Cardiology Students* and *Tickle Me Elmo Goes to the Hospital.* I kept searching. After two hours of research on all types of publication sites, I came across Dr. Wayne Sotile's *Thriving with Heart Disease.* At last! Someone had written about the victories of heart patients and was sharing it with the world. Dr. Sotile shared his years of experience treating cardiac patients and discussed their behavior in his book. I found it comforting that someone had actually observed people dealing with congestive heart failure and immediately ordered the book.

The book arrived right on schedule, and I had an entire week to read it before returning to work. It was the first book that had the words, "thriving" and "heart disease" in the same sentence. I immediately went to the index and looked up the dreaded "congestive heart failure" topic. Dr. Sotile had written a few pages on it. He wrote that CHF was usually a terminal diagnosis, but that a small percentage of patients did manage to recover and get better. He explained that a patient's recovery from CHF often depended upon many factors such as their age, ethnicity, and stress levels. He also believed that the patient's positive or negative attitude toward their treatment could influence their chances of survival. At last, someone was giving me the straight story on my new condition.

I read the book within a day and decided to call Dr. Sotile's office to thank him personally. His perky office assistant answered his phone. She explained that Dr. Sotile was on a book tour and would not be able to return calls for a month. I thanked her and asked her to relay my gratitude to him for his positive book. I told her it gave me the mustard seed of hope I needed to fight my CHF. I could hear her choking up a bit on the other end as we continued our conversation.

I tried to buoy her spirits by telling her that every pamphlet I had received on CHF from the health care teams was extremely depressing. I told her that my least favorite patient brochure was a glossy print handout called, "Living with Heart Failure." I chuckled into the phone saying, "You are not going to believe this, but it has two eighty-year-olds smiling on the cover. They remind me of Grandpa Joe and Grandma Josephine from Roald Dahl's *Charlie and the Chocolate Factory*." She giggled and thanked me for my call.

I was determined to produce something better for people who were fighting this illness. A few of them were winning their fight against heart failure, and I wanted to be one of them.

The alternative of giving up and losing the CHF battle was not acceptable to me. I had two young daughters and a husband to live for, and I was going to survive or die trying.

The next lesson I learned as a transplant patient is that you must find the resources you need, even if you have to look hard for them. An informed patient is better equipped to battle heart disease than one who is not. Patient knowledge is power.

5

DR. EGO

AFTER ONE MONTH OF TREATMENT, I learned that the first doctor I had seen in the hospital was going on a "World Medical Mission" to India and that I would need to find another cardiologist. His patient roster had been transferred to another in-network cardiologist whom I referred to as Dr. Ego. He was a short, bald man who oozed arrogance from his pores.

At my first new patient consultation with Dr. Ego, he arrived ninety minutes late from an emergency in the catheterization lab. He flung open the door to the exam room, walking in with bloody scrubs and holding out a pudgy hand. "I am Dr. Ego. And you are a very sick girl."

I immediately disliked him and jokingly replied, "No. I am a very sick Dr. Calvet." He did not find this amusing. From then on, I used my "doctor" title from my PhD in Education whenever encountering medical doctors who were arrogant. At least it put us on the same level in terms of respect when they spoke to me in a condescending manner.

After looking at my chart, he avoided eye contact with me and stared at the light fixture. "Your heart is very enlarged. The best we can do is to use medication to make it pump better. I am going to put you on some *Coreg* and we will see what happens." Within three minutes, he had made his diagnosis and left the room. I suddenly yearned for the hospital cardiologist again. At least he had taken his time speaking with me in the hospital.

Dr. Ego's nurse practitioner Gwen was more sympathetic. She must have been used to dealing with his lack of patient empathy. She explained that *Coreg* was a new cardiac drug that had positively impacted patients with heart failure. When I pressed her for details, she replied, "One-third of patients get better on the Coreg, another third stays the same, and unfortunately, the remaining third of patients gets worse." I prayed I would be in the "improved third" patient category.

Looking at the mirrored wall next to me, I saw a tired-looking woman of thirty-nine with a bluish complexion staring back. I did not like those odds. It was almost as if my intuition was telling me I would be in the bottom third who got worse. Unfortunately, this self-fulfilling prophecy would come true in the next few months.

Coreg was a very new drug at the time. When I researched it, its full name was Carvedilol and that it was classified as a "Beta Blocker," which helped the weakened heart to pump blood and fluids more effectively throughout the patient's body. Its main uses were to treat high blood pressure and heart failure. As I picked up my prescription, I hoped that it would work for me. Upon opening the box and reading the possible side effects, I became horrified. The drug patient information materials contained the words, "Cardiomyopathy can result in eventual patient death," at least ten times in large letters. This was not exactly what I wanted to read. I realized I did not have much of a choice other than to take the drugs and hope for the best.

My next appointment with Dr. Ego's clinic was a month later for an echocardiogram test. An echocardiogram is an ultrasound of the patient's heart using a Doppler radar. It looks like a Peter Max painting, with many bright colors in reds, blues, yellows, and oranges. It is similar to a baby ultrasound but with no happy bundle of joy at the end. The echocardiogram shows the anatomy of the heart in three-dimensional imaging and measures how well blood is being pumped through the heart. It is done by a cardiology technician and read by a cardiologist.

I reported to the Cardiology Lab at 10:00 a.m. The technician was kind and right on time. I spent about forty minutes having goo spread on my sternum and the roller ball rubbed back and forth across my chest. The exam bed shifted uncomfortably as the wand moved around, and I flinched. The tech looked over at me saying, "Don't worry, we are doing it right." It was annoying but not painful. I kept watching the technician's face for signs of good or bad news about my heart's condition. She had developed a poker face for her work, and I could not tell anything from her expressions. Thankfully, I would meet with Dr. Ego a week later to review the results. This was my introduction to diagnostic cardiology tests. Little did I know that I would have hundreds of them on my road to transplantation.

The next week crawled on until the day before the appointment. At last, Dr. Ego's office called to confirm. His scheduling nurse with a robotic voice called my cell phone. In a clipped tone, she said, "I am sorry, but the doctor has decided to go on a family vacation, and you will need to wait another month before he reads your results. He does not refer his patients to other doctors during his absences. May I reschedule you now?"

I was stunned. "No," I replied. "I'm finding another practice." Then I hung up. Dr. Ego's last-minute vacation plans seemed to take priority over his sick patients. I had endured enough and was ready to look for a better physician.

As with most things in life, I found my next doctor through networking. I had gone back to my job as an associate vice chancellor at the private university where I worked. For the most part, I kept my illness to myself. I did not want my colleagues to perceive me as weak or unable to do my job. I found that even providing the smallest amount of detail with a chronic illness often turned into what I refer to as "freak show questioning." During freak show questioning, people you do not really know ask you for information on your very personal medical condition. In my experience, they are usually just curious about what you are suffering from. After years of dealing with the freak show crowd, I advise patients I visit to keep their personal details of their condition to themselves. Sharing all the details of one's condition with others often results in a plethora of unwelcome opinions and ideas. It can also wear you out emotionally.

Because of these types of people, my husband and I made a pact to only discuss my medical issues with a very small, intimate group of friends and family. This included not posting on social media, which worked well for us. When my husband had news to share with this inner circle, he posted updates on a website called *Caring Bridge.* The Caring Bridge website is free of charge and was a lifesaver for us. It requires an access code provided by the patient or family to access current updates on the patient's condition. It helped our family to control the information we posted and kept worried relatives and close friends informed when we did not want to share things with the world of Facebook and other media sites. I highly recommend it to the patients I now visit as part of my volunteer work.

In a surprising turn of events, I found myself sharing my story one day with my boss, our university chancellor, whom I worked very closely with on academic initiatives. One day, he looked worn and drawn. When I asked him if something was wrong, he told me his wife was suffering from a heart condition. I made a split-second decision to tell him about my diagnosis. I also shared my frustration with him about not being able to find a good, caring cardiologist.

Without hesitating for a moment, the chancellor reached across his desk and held my hand. He said, "You need to see my wife's doctor. She is fantastic. I will use my connections to see if I can get you an appointment." This referral was an amazing gift. Our university's headquarters were situated directly across from the world-class Scripps Green Hospital in La Jolla, California, which is often referred to as "the Mayo Clinic of the West." Now I would have the opportunity to be seen by a world-class female cardiologist. My hopes soared.

The chancellor explained to me that his beloved wife was having heart valve problems. Most cardiology patients will experience one of two types of problems. The first type is what lay people call "plumbing issues." This refers to problems with the heart valves and the patient's blood flow going through the heart. The second type is "electrical issues" which refers to the rhythms and beats that run through the heart like a current. I was experiencing both electrical and plumbing issues. My CHF was causing my heart to not pump blood (plumbing) which then resulted in my heart having arrhythmias (irregular heartbeats — electrical).

Some days when I would experience arrhythmias, my beats per minute would soar up to 230 or more. This resulted in an intense fluttering of the heart, and I often felt like a hummingbird with the beats reaching astoundingly rapid levels. While the medication helped, the arrhythmias kept happening to me at a frightening rate.

I received a call from the new doctor's office the next day.

Her name was Dr. Mimi, and she ran the Center for Integrative Medicine at Scripps Clinic in La Jolla, California. The chancellor could afford the best care in the world for his wife. I was grateful that he generously helped me to get the same level of world-class treatment. I set up an appointment with Dr. Mimi the following week. Once again, I felt a slight glimmer of hope. Perhaps she could provide me with the treatment I needed to live with my CHF.

The next lesson I learned as a heart transplant patient is to network through all of your connections to find the best cardiac care you can afford. If you have connections to get the best care, use them.

6

DR. MIMI

UPON ARRIVING at Dr. Mimi's office, I noticed it was a very different place from the usual clinical settings I had visited. The signs pointed to the "lounge area" for the patient treatment waiting room in the Center. It was like a spa in Palm Springs with a New Age, calming effect. Soft Celtic music flowed from the sound system, and the medical staff wore asymmetrical pale pink cassocks instead of the usual scrubs or white lab coats. Water trickled softly from the multiple fountains placed around the lobby. Oil diffusers wafted in the air with scents of orange, lavender, and rosemary. It felt like some kind of ethereal gathering place . . . not a cardiologist's office.

A young woman with long blond hair and striking blue eyes greeted me. "Hello, Darla. I am Gretchen. We are expecting you. Please get comfortable in the lounge area and one of our care coordinators will take you back in a few moments." Gretchen was a serene European beauty who radiated peacefulness. Just looking at her made me feel awkward in my stiff work suit and heels. Shortly after taking a seat, an attractive older woman in her sixties with platinum silver hair approached me and introduced herself as Carmen, the nurse practitioner. She ushered me to a private room which was comfortable but still held the ordinary diagnostic cardiology equipment. There was no way to make scopes and machines look New Age.

Within five minutes, Dr. Mimi entered the suite. She shook my hand energetically and said, "Welcome, Darla." She was a petite, physically fit woman. She looked to be about forty years old and had a reassuring, energetic presence.

"You know," she said, "heartbeats are strange. Sometimes, they can be indicators of other issues masquerading in disguise."

"I'm not sure I follow you," I replied.

To put me at ease, she told me a cute story about another cardiac patient. A very lonely woman in her eighties was seeing Doctor Mimi for heart problems. The tests did not reveal any conditions, but the woman continued to complain about a hollow aching in her chest. After consulting with a colleague, Dr. Mimi whipped out a prescription pad during one of the woman's visits and wrote the words "One Small Dog" under the RX section. When the woman asked her about this crazy prescription, Dr. Mimi kindly replied, "You do not need drugs or surgery. You need a little friend who will keep you company and take you outside to walk. I am prescribing one small dog as a pet for that purpose." Within a week, the woman got a Yorkie puppy. She never had to be treated again as a patient at the clinic, although she is a good friend of everyone in the office. For this and many reasons, I liked Dr. Mimi. I also learned that very often, cardiac issues can be tied to the mental state of the patient.

After several minutes Dr. Mimi said, "You were so young when you got this — only thirty-nine. I would like to have you checked for sleep apnea. It may be the real cause of your problems here and not a heart condition. I want you to get a sleep study. It may be as simple as having you sleep with a CPAP device at night. Perhaps that will eliminate the concern over potential cardiac issues."

At this point in my treatment, the Coreg medication had increased my ejection fraction (EF) but only by only a few points. Ejection Fraction is defined by the American Heart Association as the key measurement, expressed as a percentage, of how much blood the left ventricle pumps out with each contraction. An ejection fraction of 60 percent means that 60 percent of the total amount of blood in the left ventricle is pushed out with each heartbeat. The higher the EF is, the better your heart is pumping. While admitted to the hospital, my EF was below normal — forty-one, to be exact. The Coreg medication had only raised it to forty-three, which indicated that my heart might not experience normal EF function again.

I immediately liked Dr. Mimi's demeanor and the fact that she did not jump to conclusions about my condition. She wanted to rule out all possibilities of causation before declaring that heart disease was my true problem. Her integrated approach was fresh and inspiring. She was looking for non-surgical, non-invasive ways to treat the problem instead of a textbook approach. I agreed to have a sleep study and walked happily back to her receptionist to make an appointment for a recheck with Dr. Mimi in a month. For the first time in the year since my diagnosis, I felt hopeful about dealing with my CHF.

Following Dr. Mimi's request, I arranged to have a sleep study the following week.

Unfortunately, the sleep study was not going to be located in the Center for Integrative Medicine. Instead, I was sent to a sleep lab clinic in Scripps Hospital. There was no calming music here — only stark white rooms that looked nothing like a place I had any desire to sleep in. I showed up at 10:30 on the night of my appointment, hoping for the best.

I was greeted by two burly technicians who had the demeanor of exhausted truckers. They walked me into the "sleep suite" and threw a hideous green hospital gown at me. "Put this on, then one of us will be in to tape you up," said the one in charge. I looked up and saw huge cameras suspended from the ceiling above. There was a glass partition on one of the walls where the techs would sit and conduct the study. I thought about bolting for the nearest exit but decided against it.

One of the technicians returned to the room with a container of thick white paste like school glue in one hand and a bunch of electrodes with leads in the other. I gripped my blanket from home and tried to stay calm. The tech smeared the white paste all over my head, attaching at least a hundred electrodes to my skull, neck, chest, and abdomen.

Do they really expect me to sleep like this? I thought.

I asked the tech what would happen if I could not get to sleep. He let out a quiet laugh, saying, "Then you get to come back and do this all again, so I would try to sleep if I were you."

The tech got me fully wired, then left the room. The other one came in and asked, "Do you have any questions?"

I replied sheepishly, "I guess I just wonder what you guys will be measuring?"

He told me they were looking for information on my sleep cycles and how many times I might stop breathing each night.

I just wanted to be back home in my own bed. They turned off the lights and I heard the cameras whirring. I rolled over on one side and lay awake until 2:00 a.m.

Miraculously, I managed to lose consciousness and sleep for a few hours. After waking up at 6:00 a.m., I was very happy to learn that the team had enough data and I could return home.

Two weeks later, I returned to the warm cocoon of Dr. Mimi's office. I hoped that sleep apnea was the true diagnosis of my problem and that I could avoid undergoing more cardiac tests. Once again, Dr. Mimi entered the room, although she did not make eye contact with me this time. "I've looked at your sleep study results," she said. "You do not have sleep apnea as I had hoped. I am not a device cardiologist, and your heart may require one to be implanted. I can confirm that your heart is very enlarged and that you do have a serious cardiac condition."

Finally looking at me, she saw the disappointment in my eyes. "I want to send you to see a colleague of mine who I think can help you. He is a cardiologist and runs the Congestive Heart Failure Recovery Clinic at Scripps. He is a specialist with medical devices that help patients get better."

As I left Dr. Mimi's office, my mind whirled. I had progressed from a regular cardiologist to a specialist, and from prescription drugs to possible devices. I was not feeling especially excited about this next round of doctor appointments. Worst of all, I had to say goodbye to Dr. Mimi.

The next lesson I learned as a heart transplant patient is that in the world of cardiology, there are many types of cardiac specialists, and you must find the right one who can treat your particular condition.

7

DR. TOM, A.K.A. HAWKEYE

A FEW WEEKS LATER, I returned to the Scripps Clinic to enter the Heart Failure and Recovery Center, headed by Dr. Mimi's colleague, Dr. Tom. Looking up at the gold letters on the wall, I was reassured to see the words "heart failure" and "recovery" in the same sentence. Until that point, my diagnosis of congestive heart failure felt much more like a death sentence than something from which I could recover. The clinic was bustling. The large waiting area had two check-in desks and was a beehive of activity from receptionists and medical professionals.

I checked in and took a seat, noticing my surroundings. Most patients in the waiting room looked like they were on borrowed time. I realized that I was about forty years younger than most of the other patients. The older woman next to me had a respiratory mask and oxygen attached to her. Her oxygen machine hissed every five minutes. I felt very out of place. It seemed like an appropriate time for a self-indulgent pity party. Thoughts such as *Why me, God?* and *I would rather be back in the regular life I had before I got this horrible illness* ricocheted through my head.

I was snapped back to reality by Terry, one of Dr. Tom's nurses. "Darla Calvet," she called out as she entered the lobby area.

I shot my hand up as if I were in grade school and shouted, "Here!" My over-eagerness gave one of the Vietnam Vets on the other side of the lobby a good chuckle from across the room. I had not assumed the role of the sick person by this point. I still saw myself as a temporary visitor, someone with a hall pass who was walking through the clinic but not really staying.

Nurse Terry did the usual routine, weighing me, measuring my height, and taking my vitals.

She put me into a private exam room and indicated that the doctor would be right in. I was getting used to my doctor visits. I had become bold while waiting for doctors. Terry had wisely left my file outside in the hallway. Otherwise, I would have snooped. No one had really leveled with me at this time about how sick I truly was or how much longer I might have remained on the planet. I hoped that Dr. Tom would be the one to provide me with these truthful answers.

There was a soft knock at the door, and it opened slowly. The first time I saw Dr. Tom, I thought of Alan Alda's character Hawkeye on the famous M-A-S-H television show. He was tall, gray, handsome, and very charming. More importantly, he had twinkling blue eyes and a sense of humor. My first impression after meeting him was that *he cared about his patients.*

After running the usual in-office tests, he sighed. I asked him, "How bad is it? I am tired of everyone treating me like I cannot deal with the truth. Please tell me."

Dr. Tom sat down on the stool in front of the exam bed and rolled up next to me. He took both of my hands in his and looked me straight in the eyes. "It is not great. Your heart is very enlarged and not pumping too well. But I will tell you this. I can make you better. We will make you well. My goal is to have you die a happy grandmother at the age of eighty-eight, in your sleep or surrounded by your grandkids. We cannot have you die now; you're too young. We can do this."

I wept tears of relief. Dr. Tom was the first physician to give me this much hope. He was honest. He explained to me that with heart failure, there are three sequential phases of treatment. The first phase of treatment involved prescribing medications. He explained that while they could be effective, the body could become used to them over time, and they could lose their effectiveness. They did not cure heart failure, he explained. Instead, these drugs maximized the way my heart would beat to get more blood throughout the body. He concurred with Dr. Ego's choice of Coreg as my main medication. He said it was the best Beta Blocker available for CHF patients at the time.

Dr. Tom then explained the second phase of heart failure treatment — mechanical devices. With my overactive imagination, I immediately pictured myself as part android. He told me about a new external heart pump called a Left Ventricular Assist Device (LVAD). I would eventually become the thirteenth person implanted with an LVAD at Scripps Memorial Hospital in La Jolla in 2013, when they were first becoming available. Dr. Tom said that for the time being, medications appeared to be the best treatment option for my tired and overworked heart.

"What's the third treatment option?" I asked Dr. Tom.

"Well, you're not there yet, but it is the organic solution of transplant," he responded. He gave me a visual description of how he viewed all of his congestive heart failure patients: "I think of all of my patients being at an outdoor picnic, somewhere with cliffs like Torrey Pines in La Jolla Cove. Some of them are sitting down, eating their lunch with their families. Those are my patients treated with medications. Others are edging closer to the cliff and require medical devices. Some are on the edge of the cliff, and they require a transplant." This simple explanation of CHF made things very clear. With Dr. Tom's permission, I have shared it with many patients.

Dr. Tom's kind demeanor was no coincidence. Several years after being treated by him, I learned that he had enrolled in the seminary to become a priest before entering medical school. His kindness and stellar treatment of patients made complete sense to me after learning about his past. Dr. Tom eventually became not only my lead cardiologist but a true patient advocate and friend. Without him and his staff, I doubt I would still be alive. Finding the right cardiologist to treat your heart condition is just that vital. It can make the difference in one's survival. Dr. Tom communicated with my insurance company, advocated for the best specialists to be on my care team, and literally saved my life multiple times. During a fight with heart disease, you must have at least one medical champion in your corner. Dr. Tom was my champion and still manages my treatment to this day.

Dr. Tom and his nurse practitioner, Laura, treated me effectively for eight years with medication. During this time, the Coreg and diuretics did their job to keep the blood and fluids moving around my body effectively. I had to be near the bathroom at all times, taking more than eight doses of diuretics a day to fight my ongoing cardiac edema.

More importantly, his entire staff walked the lonely and difficult road of CHF treatment by my side. They were no longer just medical professionals: they were our extended family members and advocates.

We shared some good laughs along the way, too. I

remember one office visit while I was sitting in the lobby during the holidays. *The Grinch Who Stole Christmas* was playing on one of the television monitors. After I got back into the exam room, I looked at Laura and Dr. Tom saying, "You know, I am just like the Grinch . . . my heart did grow two sizes in one day!" We all had a good laugh and went on with the day's visit.

Despite the team's heroic efforts, my CHF did not improve. I was one of the unlucky 30 percent of patients who continued to get worse despite medication treatment. My body retained high amounts of water despite the diuretics. Even worse, my arrhythmias were wilder than a percussion session. They were also very dangerous. One of the key reasons people die from heart failure is due to heart attack or stroke caused by these highly irregular electric rhythms. The American Heart Association defines an arrhythmia as any change from the normal sequence of electrical impulses. The electrical impulses may happen too fast, too slowly, or erratically, causing the heart to beat out of rhythm.

Dr. Tom also explained to me that my Ejection Fraction (EF) had begun dropping since my last visit, from forty-three to thirty-nine. When I first saw Dr. Tom in 2005, my EF was classified as low normal at forty-one. A normal range is defined as between forty and sixty by the American Heart Association. If you are a CHF patient, the EF is your life-or-death measurement. By the time I had been treated by Dr. Tom for six years, the drugs were clearly losing their treatment influence on my body.

Each echocardiogram revealed a sinking EF. In 2008, my EF had dropped to a very low twenty-five. The arrhythmias were increasing as my overworked heart tried to push itself even harder. Things were looking pretty grim. I often found myself short of breath and unable to walk more than a few feet, which frustrated me since I was used to being physically active and mobile. Depression began to set in as my health declined.

During one of my regular visits, Dr. Tom once again held my hands. He said, "The drugs do not seem to be working anymore, twinkle toes. Our best option is to have you see our surgeon and to have him put an AICD in." The full name for an AICD is an Automatic Implantable Cardioverter-Defibrillator. It is a device designed to monitor the patient's heartbeat. This device can deliver an electrical impulse or shock to the heart when it senses a life-threatening change in the heart's rhythm. It is usually implanted with a pacemaker, which monitors the pacing of one's heart. Dr. Tom handed me a referral to his surgeon friend Dr. John, and I officially entered the second phase of cardiac treatment — medical device implantation.

The next lesson I learned as a heart transplant patient is that a good doctor will treat you to the best of his or her ability, then refer you to more specialists as they are needed. Your treatment plan, health, and welfare should always come first.

8

DR. JOHN AND SPARKY

WITHIN A MONTH, I sat in Dr. John's consultation room, nervously flipping through old magazines. It was 2012. The October 2008 issue of *People* I held in my hands featured a close-up photo of Kanye West and Kim Kardashian with the word "Dating!" running across it. I had never had any type of major surgery before. The thought of having a device implanted in my chest made me nauseous with fear.

The office nurse called my name, and I was taken to a small exam room. I looked around and saw plastic models of the heart with defibrillators and electrical lead wires protruding from them. They were branded with cardiac medical device companies' logos. I wondered if I could pretend I was a lost patient and leave the room without being noticed.

There was a quick knock at the door, and Dr. John entered the exam room, smiling. He stretched out his giant, non-surgeon-like paw and gave my hand a firm shake. He was about six feet tall, with a stocky, football player build. He was tan and looked like he had just returned from a few weeks in the Hamptons. He plopped down on the impossibly small stool in the room and looked over my chart and vitals. Glancing down at me, he said, "Dr. Tom has the right idea about giving you an AICD implant. He and I are good friends, you know. I have implanted quite a few of his patients."

Dr. John grabbed one of the plastic heart models and showed me the AICD unit and how it worked. It was about the size of a pat of butter. It was made out of titanium steel and had multiple leads emerging from it. For some reason, the wildly protruding leads reminded me of a sea creature I had seen in the tide pools as a young child. The most amazing thing about the AICD was that it was a miniature version of the large defibrillator units that are seen at airports and other public places. All of that technology was going to be surgically implanted into my ailing heart. It was a lot for me to take in psychologically. And it was another version of what psychologists call "the patient's 'new normal'" or changed state of physical and mental being. Having this device would help me to stay alive — but it would also shock me over thirty times and change the way my everyday life had been for forty years. I had an overwhelming sense of dread as I heard all the details about the upcoming implant surgery.

While I was not happy about becoming implanted, I was relieved that it would help to alleviate my 230 beats per minute hummingbird heart arrythmias. When I asked Dr. John what it would feel like if the defibrillator launched, he replied, "Well, some of my patients say it feels like being kicked in the chest by a mule. The shock lasts only a second, then you recover, and your heart slows down. I cannot tell you what it feels like because I have never had one." Dr. John was the first physician to admit to me as a patient that while doctors are medical experts, they cannot give you the user perspective on interventional therapies. Only patients can help other patients to truly understand what they will go through with medication, devices, and transplant.

At this point, I realized I could ask other patients about their experience . . . if I could find them.

One of the hardest things about being a cardiac patient is finding your tribe for help. Knowing that someone has walked in your footsteps and survived has a huge, positive effect on one's outlook about your treatment. I quickly began making calls to try to find a patient support group in my local San Diego area. These are usually offered by local hospitals and cardiac teams and can offer solid support to those who are dealing with chronic cardiac illness. As I now tell patients, *your vibe is your tribe.*

The morning of the first implant surgery was fairly uneventful. While I was nervous, I accepted it as the next phase of my treatment. I was the second surgical case of the morning and reported to the hospital at 6:00 a.m. It would be the first of many heart surgeries for me. The regular course of pre-surgery events took place that morning. The nurses prepped me for the surgery. The anesthesiologist came and told me what to expect. Then Dr. John came in and gave me a big bear hug. He told me not to worry and that the procedure would take about an hour to complete. I had already been waiting for three hours by the time they wheeled me into the operating room.

After I woke up in the recovery room (professionally referred to as "telemetry"), I was told that I did fine during the implant. There was now a fully operating minicomputer in my chest. It was hooked up to my left ventricle with tiny plastic-coated wire leads which were inserted directly into my heart. They had also implanted my pacemaker unit, which literally kept my heart pacing at the appropriate rate. For some reason, the entire experience reminded me of an old Warner Brothers cartoon where Wile E. Coyote was shown holding a bundle of ACME dynamite. I looked down at the newly implanted defibrillator where it bulged under my skin in a perfect square. I wondered, *When will it go off for the first time? And will I end up looking like a burned coyote afterwards?* Only time would tell.

The angry slash over my left breast would eventually heal, but I had mixed feelings about being part woman and part machine. One of the hardest things for me to get my mind around was that this machine was now part of my body. I needed it to survive, and it would do its job of shocking me if my body needed it. While I was relieved that it would resuscitate me, the thought of feeling the shock voltage made me very anxious. What if it launched in a public place or while I was driving? How would I cope? I would soon experience this very event for myself.

To make light of this serious situation, I decided to nickname the device "Sparky." I had no idea how prophetic that nickname would be in the years to come. My Italian Catholic mom preferred to call it "the angel in my chest." While I admired her optimism, I did not share it. Sparky was a cougar set to pounce when my heart started beating irregularly. Living with that knowledge on a daily basis was terrifying and stressful.

A year went by without incident. At that point, Sparky was a silent watchman. Then, things began to change. It was a typical sunny San Diego day in October of 2012. I had just returned home with a friend after enduring three exhausting hours of hearing Russell Crowe trying to sing opera in the film version of *Les Misérables*. Fatigued, I laid down on our family room couch and was very light-headed. My daughter Annie, who was a high school senior then, was making a snack in the kitchen. It was 4:26 p.m.

As I lowered myself down on the couch, my vision began to blur, and I started losing consciousness. The last thing I heard Annie yell across the house to my husband was, "Mom is doing something weird on the couch! She's flopping around like a fish, Dad!" What had occurred was called a brown-out. My heart rhythm had become so faint that my defibrillator was preparing to launch. When a patient's heartbeat becomes weakened, the defibrillator will launch to put it back into a normal rhythm. Thankfully, my heart rhythm corrected itself before the launch occurred. While I was scared after this incident, I did not feel any pain. The launch had been averted . . . at least for now.

To this day, I cannot watch that version of *Les Misérables*. Too many bad memories. My family refers to it jokingly as the "dancing trout incident" due to my erratic twitching on our couch. While this may sound cruel, the humor did help us to get through these unpredictable and frightening events.

This episode left me stunned and confused. How could I even think about driving when I could pass out behind the wheel? There were many social and ethical issues arising from having a medical device that the doctors had not warned me about. I was going to encounter more of them as I lived with the AICD and pacemaker over the next six years.

After the trout dance incident on the couch, I had another follow-up appointment with Dr. John, the surgeon. The AICD has a type of memory card in its tiny computer. By placing a clear circular wand over my chest, Dr. John was able to print out all of the shockwaves that had been issued prior to the aborted launch. I stared blankly at him, trying to accept my "new normal."

Dr. John read the data then said, "I know it is difficult when the AICD goes off. But the good news is, it put your heart back into its normal rhythm without shocking you."

As much as I dreaded it, I asked, "Should I stop driving? I do not want to hurt anyone."

Dr. John's answer was clear as mud. "If you had been shocked, I would have automatically revoked your license. But since you weren't, it is up to you."

I was still working and trying to remain independent in spite of my heart problems. The loss of independence by active patients is one of the hardest things that most of us encounter as we begin to deal with our chronic illness.

The pre-shock brown-out episode had affected me so dramatically that I made my own decision to stop driving. I would not have been able to live with myself if my AICD had deployed and I had injured someone else. It is hard enough living with heart failure but knowing that you might hurt someone else is unconscionable. My husband Pat would start driving me to work in the morning. We started paying my daughter Annie a small allowance to pick me up after work. I began to feel more helpless and removed from my normal life as the CHF progressed.

The next lesson I learned as a transplant patient is that you know your body better than anyone else. If your gut tells you to do or not do something based on how you feel physically, listen to it, and take appropriate action.

9

SHOCKS AND SHAME

ON THE RARE occasions when I did go out in public, my disability was hidden from the world. Dr. John issued me a red temporary handicap placard so that I could park closer to buildings. He wanted me to walk the shortest amount possible to keep my defibrillator from going off during an arrhythmia.

On a trip to Target, my daughter Annie parked my car and we put the disability placard up. We were running into the pharmacy to pick up another prescription.

A scraggly elderly man approached the car and yelled, "You do not have a handicap! You should be ashamed of yourself!"

Keeping completely calm, I turned and pulled back my t-shirt to reveal my AICD scar. "Do you see this? I growled. "This is from heart surgery. You need to stop judging people!" He was still muttering nonsense to himself as we walked away. For the first time in my life, someone made a poor judgment about my disability, and it hurt — a lot.

One of the worst side effects of the AICD was getting cabin fever. I had been implanted for about a year when my husband

Pat tried to cheer me up by taking me to a local Octoberfest in San Diego. Although I was usually tired, I still tried to make an effort to get out and be with people. It helped me keep my sanity during the illness and alleviate some of my depression.

We drove to the Octoberfest venue and parked about a block away. We started walking, and I immediately began to feel dizzy and weak. Determined to make it to the event, I soldiered on walking. Suddenly, I heard a high-pitched whine in my ears and a mild buzz run through my veins. Then I heard a loud *POP* followed by the mule kick in my chest. The next thing I knew, I was lying flat on the ground. My AICD had shocked me in front of hundreds of people. I had flown about five feet across the grass. A small crowd gathered around me. Stunned and embarrassed, I wished the earth would swallow me up.

My husband managed to keep calm and left to get our car. There would be no brats or beer for us that night. Instead, we spent our Octoberfest date in the emergency room at Scripps Clinic in La Jolla. A shock from the AICD was an automatic ticket to the ER and hospital. While I was implanted with my AICD, I would be shocked over thirty times. It is a small miracle that I still have hair on my head. It is a bigger wonder that this hair is still straight after being shocked so many times.

Once I had experienced my first shock, some of my fears abated, but my anxiety increased. I knew what the shock would feel like, and that I would recover. What I did not know was when these shocks would take place and how severe they would be. Frequently, shocks will come in waves when the defibrillator is attempting to shock the patient's heart back into a normal rhythm. While I was grateful for the telemedicine that saved my life, it caused me the stress of dreading the next launch. It was a very confusing time for me and my family. We all felt overwhelmed living with this new technology. Worse, I felt guilty for putting them all through this adjustment.

I joined an AICD support group, which was run by a sympathetic social worker. She said, "I really wish I knew what you all are going through. I just cannot imagine . . ." While I appreciated her sense of empathy, I benefitted more from hearing other patients' experience with their defibrillators. I had so many questions. How did people live in fear of knowing that they could be shocked at any moment? Did they experience post-traumatic stress disorder as a result of living with this device? There did not seem to be a wealth of information in this area. Often, medical technology will be so new that early users must share their experiences with each other. This is why I share my story with so many patients. My goal is to let them know they are not alone in their suffering and that we have all experienced the turmoil they are going through.

Sparky seemed to have a knack for making public appearances. He launched at the grocery store, in church, at parties, and at home. The craziest launch happened after I had taken a trip to the grocery store and was loading bags into my trunk. Sparky zapped me and I flew into the trunk, landing on top of the bags. Simultaneously, another woman who was an off-duty paramedic was walking into the store and eventually pulled me out of my car trunk. She and I shared a good laugh after she realized I was all right.

The medical device company did not offer any information on how to cope with your anxiety while living with the defibrillator. Their patient materials seemed to be geared toward inactive seniors. I continued to take short walks and do gentle yoga, hoping that it would keep me in the best condition possible. The effort it took me to walk short distances indicated that my body was continuing to worsen. While the AICD was keeping me alive, it was not a long-term solution. At my next appointment with Dr. Tom, he asked how my quality of life was. I shrugged. "I'm grateful to be alive but living with this device has rocked my world in so many ways."

Dr. Tom and his team tried vigilantly to keep my spirits up. Laura, the nurse practitioner, knew that I wanted to help others. She nominated me to attend the WomenHeart National Health Coalition training at the Mayo clinic. The Mission of the WomenHeart Symposium is to improve the health and quality of life of women living with or at risk of heart disease, and to advocate for their benefit. I was accepted into the next class and flew to Minnesota to meet forty-nine other women who were battling heart disease. In the meantime, my Ejection Fraction had continued to drop to 17 percent. The scary cliff that Dr. Tom had used in his metaphor about heart patients appeared to be looming in the distance.

The next lesson I learned as a transplant patient is that while medical devices are life savers, very little is known about the psychological and social effects they have on their users. More studies are needed to help doctors and their patients learn how to deal with the social impact of these modern medical advances.

10

GO RED

THE PLANETS ALIGNED, and I was able to go to the WomenHeart Symposium at no cost. The chancellor who had referred me to Dr. Mimi generously agreed to allow me to take paid time off to travel to Minnesota to the Mayo Clinic. I was ecstatic. I realized how lucky I was to work for an employer who would be so supportive of my health and well-being. I received an okay from Dr. Tom to make my travel arrangements. While there was a chance of a launch, I was willing to take the risk of traveling to the Symposium at the Mayo Clinic in Minnesota.

WomenHeart estimates that over 96 percent of women with heart disease are misdiagnosed when they experience symptoms. I was one of them. My general practitioner dismissed my complaints of fatigue as "doing too much" between work and home life. He misdiagnosed me with asthma and prescribed a medication that could have killed me with my underlying heart condition. I soon learned at the Symposium that there were many women who had been told the same thing by their primary care physicians.

I arrived in Minnesota and checked into the hotel reserved for WomenHeart attendees. I could almost pick out the other WomenHeart participants looking around the lobby. Most of us looked permanently tired and had a blue undertone to our skin due to a lack of circulation. Some of us had thick ankles, indicating edema and heart problems. Despite all of these medical issues, we all wore big smiles on our faces as we checked in. We started to talk about our cardiac experiences and bonded immediately. We were relieved to have found our tribe of other women heart patients who were suffering with heart disease but continuing to live their best lives.

We met for an orientation dinner that evening. We were greeted with lovely gift bags that contained nightgowns, cosmetics, and books for us. Over dinner, women struck up lively conversations about their diagnoses and their treatments. We were greeted by Lisa Tate, the executive director of WomenHeart at the time. She showed us a slideshow of women in professional portraits who proudly showed their heart surgery scars to the camera. "This was our white shirt campaign," Lisa shared proudly with the group. She introduced us to some alumni of the program who had greatly benefitted from their time at the Mayo Clinic. Their stories were inspirational and motivated me to make the most of my time as a WomenHeart participant.

I was so grateful that my medical team had nominated me to attend the Symposium. It occurred to me during dinner that I had the opportunity to become a Women's Heart Health Advocate and help other women struggling with heart disease. I felt empowered for the first time since receiving my diagnosis to use my illness for positive social change for other women.

The next few days consisted of attending cardiology lectures at the Mayo Clinic and activities focusing on WomenHeart and its purpose. As a National Coalition, it was based in

Washington, D.C. Its small staff worked on getting the word out about females and heart disease. One of their key initiatives was to advocate for more federal research money to be appropriated to Women's Heart Health Initiatives. I was very proud to be a part of this group.

I enjoyed the WomenHeart experience so much that I applied as an alumna to attend their policy session institute on Capitol Hill. I was also accepted into this program and led a group of female heart patients to meet with senators and legislators to get a Women's Heart Health Bill signed and passed in the Senate. We helped to raise awareness that heart disease is the number one killer of men and women in the United States.

We met a very interesting female senator when we were seeking support for the Women's Heart Health Research Bill. The senator's sister had suffered from heart illness, yet she had not taken the time to read or sign the bill. After meeting with the members of our group and hearing our stories, she signed the bill immediately, and the funding was allocated. The impact of our small groups was mighty: our visits resulted in over two and a half million dollars being earmarked for continued research for Women's Heart Health.

One of the most interesting things I learned through my volunteer work with WomenHeart is that heart disease is not a "sexy" illness. Before my involvement with WomenHeart, I had not realized that illnesses could be sexy. A WomenHeart public relations staff member explained it this way: "All social causes fight for time in the media. There is a definite stigma to a disease from which many people do not recover. Unlike breast cancer and the 'save the tatas' campaign, there is nothing sexy about heart disease. We spent two million dollars to brand the Go Red and Red Dress campaigns. It will take years for us to know whether this investment will be a good one or not."

Here is a bit of background on the WomenHeart Go Red

Campaign. Go Red for Women is the American Heart Association's national movement to end heart disease and stroke for women. The symbol of this movement is a red dress, which is used on their promotional materials and pins. The women at my table were divided: some of them liked the Red Dress campaign, while others thought it was a tawdry, inappropriate symbol for the movement. The WomenHeart participants soon learned that marketing an illness is a very tricky thing.

Going to the WomenHeart events taught me three important things. First, that the majority of women with heart disease are misdiagnosed, as I had been during my annual physical. Second, that the road to recovery was very lonely for most of us, even though we all suffered from heart disease. Third, the best way I could help other women was to get involved, despite how I was feeling physically. Ironically, this volunteerism was the very thing I needed to get out of my own head and problems. I recommend programs such as WomenHeart, Mended Hearts, and others to all survivors who want to make positive social change for all cardiac patients. Sometimes getting out of our own heads and helping others is the best thing we can do to alleviate stress and depression.

I was lucky. When I got ill, I experienced symptoms related to my CHF. Not all heart patients are so fortunate. Dr. Helene was at an annual medical conference giving a speech. She noticed a woman in the front row who looked very pale and was swaying in her seat. The woman attempted to get up and leave the auditorium. She collapsed. Dr. Helene sprang into action conducting CPR and revived her failing heart, saving her life. Thanks to her efforts, this young woman with three children lived to see them later that evening. When we discussed this incident, Dr. Helene modestly said, "I did what any good doctor would do. For some people with CHF, death is the first symptom." For the first time during my illness, I was actually glad that I had experienced symptoms telling me how sick I had become.

The next lesson I learned as a transplant patient is that activism is the most noble and profound way to give meaning to one's illness, no matter how bad the sickness seems. For a list of resources for heart health, please see the epilogue.

11

THE GHOST AND THE MACHINE: MY LVAD JOURNEY

UPON MY RETURN from the WomenHeart trip to San Diego, I reported for my regular checkup with Dr. Tom. After running more tests, he looked concerned. "Remember when I said I didn't want you too close to that cliff?"

"Yes," I responded wearily.

"Well, despite your medical devices, you are getting very close. Your AICD keeps launching, and it is hard on your heart, which is now the size of a deflated basketball. I think you might need the support of an LVAD."

While I knew my heart had swollen, I had pictured it being more the size of a baseball than a basketball. I also knew that the LVAD was the last weapon we had available to help get me strong enough to transplant.

I asked Dr. Tom to explain to me in laymen's terms what an LVAD was. The LVAD acronym stands for "Left Ventricular Assist Device." Dr. Tom explained that an LVAD is a Ventricular Assist Device (VAD) — also known as a mechanical circulatory support device. Its function is to help pump blood from the lower chambers of your heart (ventricles) to the rest of your body.

He then pointed to the poster on the exam room wall. It was created by Thoratec Inc., the company that manufactured the LVAD. It depicted a grandfatherly-type male model (who was somehow still attractive), wearing a device strapped around his midsection. An inset cartoon showed the mechanics of how the LVAD worked as an external heart pump.

"How long has this thing been around?" I asked.

"For about a year," Dr. Tom said. "It is new, but the technology is really helping people. I just want you to go home and consider it. I know it will be a big life change for you."

I knew immediately that the "big life change" would not necessarily be pleasant.

I sat in the exam room, stunned at the amount of technology that was going to be placed into my ailing body. Dr. Tom saw the distress on my face. He explained, "The LVAD is the brainchild of an engineer and a cardio-thoracic surgeon. It is relatively new but has been very positive in treating late-stage cardiomyopathy patients. It weighs eight and a half pounds and is an external heart pump that is attached to your body by a drive line that goes through your abdomen. It costs a million dollars to be surgically implanted, but it could really improve your quality of life." When I asked Dr. Tom how many people he had implanted the LVAD in, he looked away. "We have done an LVAD surgery on about ten people. It is a relatively new surgical treatment. I know it is hard for you to think about, but I believe it will save your life."

I felt queasy while I looked around the treatment room at the new and strange device in the drawing. I had been a swimmer since I could crawl. The LVAD would change that. There would be no submerging in water once this million-dollar piece of life-saving equipment was installed into my body. Not even baths were permitted. The device, plus its two lithium batteries that were the size of small notebooks, would need to be attached to my body at all times. At night, the machine would be plugged into a recharging unit. The LVAD could give me better health, but what about all the other effects of daily living with a mechanical heart device? I needed time to think all of this over.

One of the staff nurses explained to me that there are two types of LVAD patients. The first group is known as "destination therapy patients." These people are not eligible for transplant and wear LVADs for the remainder of their lives. The second group of people are known as "bridging patients," who wear their LVADs until their bodies grow strong enough to be transplanted. The pump takes the place of regular heartbeats and helps blood and fluids move through the body, aiding in respiration and other functions. Dr. Tom had told me that at forty-nine, I should be able to qualify for eventual transplant. I was grateful to be in the second group of LVAD users who were bridging to transplant.

In the end, I did not choose when my LVAD would be installed. An emergency surgery was done when my heart had almost stopped beating and the choice was made for me by my medical team due to my failing body. Despite Dr. Tom's and Dr. John's best efforts, we were running out of time and options. My body had become completely backed up with fluids. One evening as I was preparing dinner for my family, I noticed water seeping from my legs and feet, which was pooling on the kitchen floor. To my shock and dismay, the massive cardiac edema in my body had nowhere to go but through my skin! Despite the medications and devices, I was literally drowning in the fluids my heart could not pump through my body. I knew it was time to get help. That night, I reluctantly agreed to go to Dr. Tom's clinic the next day to show him how bad my condition had become.

The following day in the clinic, my appearance must have been horrifying for the staff. The normally chipper nurses were somber and alarmed when they saw me walking toward the clinic with huge swollen ankles, a bluish complexion, and no energy. Jocelyn, one of my favorite nurses, put her arm around me and said, "Okay honey, let's go really slow and easy now. One step at a time. Into the exam room, please." She would later tell me that my appearance was so frightening she needed to go into the staff room to calm herself down and stop crying.

Dr. Tom was on a much-needed family vacation, so Nurse Practitioner Laura attended to me. She breezed into the exam room, took a look at me, and stopped dead in her tracks. "I am going to call the doctor in Mexico. You are in bad shape. We need to admit you to the hospital, stat." I knew at that moment that I would not be returning home for a long time.

I sat in silence for the next ten minutes in the cold exam room. I shook my head violently in anger and cursed at myself. I had done everything my team asked me to do. I had taken my meds, eaten healthy foods, rested, and reduced my workload. The CHF was winning my fight for life, and none of it seemed fair or logical. I had dealt with the illness for almost ten years. I was tired and discouraged but refused to give up. My daughters had not even graduated from college yet. I had family to live for and a reason to keep going. Dr. Tom agreed with Nurse Laura on the phone that I needed to be admitted immediately.

When he returned from his vacation a few days later, Dr. Tom called Dr. Sam, the cardio-thoracic surgeon who installed the LVADs at Scripps Hospital in La Jolla. They had a very serious discussion about how the LVAD surgery would be needed to save my life. The cardiac nurses would later tell me that when Dr. Tom and Dr. Sam worked with the hospital social worker, who made multiple calls to my insurance company. Dr. Sam was a very famous cardio thoracic surgeon whom I was lucky to have on my team. They insisted that I receive the LVAD surgery immediately. At one point, Dr. Tom walked the halls of his clinic shouting, "SHE CANNOT DIE. NOT ON MY WATCH!" I cannot help but think that his tenacity and advocacy saved my life. I will always be grateful for the fight these doctors endured on my behalf to get me the treatment I needed to live.

Meanwhile, I had been admitted to the hospital by Dr. Tom's team and was trying to be hopeful about my treatment. As I was being settled into my hospital room, I felt extremely weak. The orderly on duty tossed me a hospital gown and instructed me to change. My mom had been visiting us and sat in the corner of the small hospital room, looking forlorn and helpless. My husband's office was conveniently located across the street from the hospital, and he was on his way over to meet us.

As I tried to make my way into the hospital bathroom, I pitched forward and held my hand on the end of the hospital bed to steady myself. I had been to this hospital many times, but somehow this visit felt especially ominous. I thought to myself, "Easy girl, you don't want to pass out." As I stood up slowly, my feet went out from under me, the room turned black, and I lost consciousness. I did not know before losing consciousness that it would be more than two months before I woke up again.

The next lesson I learned as a transplant patient is: If your condition gets worse, do not wait to get help. Your life could depend on how quickly you get treatment. When you are in doubt, go directly to the clinic or to the hospital for medical treatment.

12

WHILE YOU WERE SLEEPING

EXACTLY SIXTY-TWO DAYS after I had fainted in the Scripps Green hospital room, I woke up in complete darkness. My heart raced. I had no idea where I was or what happened to me since I passed out on the day I was admitted. I was unable to see without my contacts or glasses and tried to speak but could not emit a sound. For those first few moments, I thought perhaps maybe I was in some kind of purgatory and that this was my eternal bus stop. I felt a distinct heaviness as I tried to move my legs. I felt down around my abdomen and detected the LVAD unit, with a drive line going through my abdomen and its two large lithium batteries attached to my body. The LVAD surgery had occurred. But when, why, and how had it happened? I sat in darkness, vainly searching for the remote control and the button to call the night shift nurse.

I felt a weird combination of relief and confusion. I could decipher from the blurry digits on the clock that it was about 4:00 a.m. I had no idea what day, month, or year it was. I knew from the LVAD installation that some time must have passed, but how much? I must have woken up during a skeletal night shift with very few nurses in the hospital unit. I swung my head as far around as I could, only to see the outlines and lights of seventeen machines in the room, all helping to keep me alive. I immediately started to panic. I seemed to be more machine than human with all of the leads and tubes running in and out of my body. I was also intubated and unable to speak, which was terrifying. I could discern from the many machines attached to me that I was also in the Cardiac Intensive Care Unit, known as the CICU. This was where the gravely ill cardiac patients were sent by their teams.

"Stay calm," I told myself. Someone had to be around . . . somewhere. The heavy blackout curtains were drawn around my glass cube room, making me feel claustrophobic. After a long wait, the curtains were flung open by Patricia, my morning nurse, who was starting her shift. She smiled sweetly, saying, "Oh, good. You are awake. We have been waiting for you to wake up." I was confused and had no idea how I had arrived at my current state in the hospital bed. At that time, the CICU was located in the basement of the Scripps Green Hospital Facility, next to the morgue. It was not exactly a cheery place. I heard some orderlies joking to each other that it was "death's waiting room."

Realizing that I could not speak, Patricia took my hand and spoke softly, "You are okay. You have been in a medically induced coma for over two months. During that time, we needed to perform emergency open heart surgery and save your life by installing the LVAD, which you have probably noticed is attached to your body." I shuddered and pulled the sheets up around my neck. God only knew how close I had come to death. I was about to find out.

To say that I was disorientated is a massive understatement. While I knew I had been at death's door, I had no idea of the massive effort and heartbreaking decisions that went into saving my life by my doctors, nurses, and family members. I kept looking at things around the room. There were cards, messages from friends, and several prayer bracelets that had been put on both of my wrists. Patricia looked at me saying, "Take it easy. Your husband will be coming over today to visit you. Try not to talk. It will strain your trachea, and you are intubated, so you really cannot speak anyway. I will be back soon to bring you your breakfast."

I sat in stunned silence as I watched Patricia leave the room. My hand clenched at my throat, and I realized there was a large plastic tube which had been inserted from my mouth and throat down into esophagus and chest.

I still remember the view from Room 5 in the CICU. I spent a good deal of time there, both conscious and unconscious. It occurred to me that I was probably one of the sickest patients, given that I was close enough to the nurses' station to see it through the door from my bed. I could even read the nurses' bulletin board, which had a flyer entitled "Avoiding Sexual Harassment" posted on it. A person notices little things like that when they are confined to an ICU hospital bed 24/7, with only one view straight ahead. There was a tiny window at the back of the room that showed a rectangle of blue sky above the parking lot. Besides my bed and the machines, there was one large reclining chair and a mounted television that received three channels. This would be my home for the next two months of recovery.

While I was very grateful and relieved to be alive, I thought of my family. How had my husband coped during my absence with our two young adult girls? How had they dealt with this horrible situation? My eldest, Claire, was a high school senior. My youngest, Annie, was now a high school freshman. It made me sad to think about missing the important events that were going on in their young lives.

My next thought was my job. What had happened to it? Had someone finally disclosed how sick I had been while continuing to work? It gave me pause to consider that this had happened during my absence. I did not know that my husband had requested a one-year leave of absence after I fainted at the hospital. I was grateful he did this on my behalf. During my last days at my job, my ego kept me from seeking support even as I struggled to walk a few hundred feet from the parking lot to the elevator up to my office.

A few moments later, Nurse Patricia returned with my "breakfast." It was a peach colored container of liquid protein that looked like cement. I watched in awe as she said, "Down the hatch" and poured it into my feeding tube. "Can you taste anything?" she asked. I shook my head "no." The only sensation I felt was the cold sludge making its way down the feeding tube in the back of my throat. I had lost quite a bit of weight during my two-month nap. Thirty-four pounds to be exact. My body, which had always been very muscular, was now atrophied and weak.

The LVAD was the third device to be surgically placed into my body after the AICD defibrillator and pacemaker. It cost over a million dollars to install. Now, my job of learning to live with it began. There would be no swimming in the near future. The eight pounds of life-saving state-of-the-art medical equipment that was now part of my body would require ongoing care. I had no idea at that time the battles that had taken place to get the LVAD device installed. I would have certainly died without it.

The next lesson I learned as a transplant patient is: Your medical team must fight to save your life. Even with your insurance company. You do not have the luxury of time on your side.

13

LIFE IN THE CICU AS LUCKY NUMBER THIRTEEN

MY FIRST CONSCIOUS day in the CICU seemed like a month. I was too incapacitated to get out of bed. I lay awake, watching hours of poor-quality television programs. I saw an episode of the old *Bewitched* television show from the early 1970s. *Oh, the days of striped bell bottom pants and good old Endora,* I mused. My life was much simpler when I was a child in the '70s. Except for visitors, I had lost most of my connectivity with the outside world. The CICU did not allow patients to have working cell phones and ensured that they would not be used by blocking us access to the internet connection. After three hours on day one, I started to feel like a caged lion. I looked at the giant industrial clock on the wall. It was only 11:05 a.m.

Around 3:30 in the afternoon, my husband Pat came bounding through the doors of the CICU with a big smile on his face. He entered my room and shouted, "You are awake! Finally!"

The nurses had left a laminated card on my patient tray to help me communicate by spelling out words since I could not speak. I felt like a circus pony that was trying to count for spectators by pounding its hoof. Pat asked me how I was doing, and I shakily spelled out the words, "O-K-A-Y" on the card. It was very frustrating to have to communicate by pointing to letters and spelling words like a young child.

Pat leaned over the bed and looked me in the eye. Slowly and compassionately, he began to tell me the story of what had transpired over the last few months. "The *Reader's Digest* version of how you got here is this. You passed out in your hospital room. You remember that, right?" I slowly nodded in agreement. "Well, after that, you got really bad with irregular heartbeats. They had to transfer you to a bigger hospital, and you flatlined. We almost lost you, Darla. They revived you back to life with the paddles, and Dr. Tom and Dr. Sam decided that they were going to install you with an LVAD that night in an effort to save your life. The surgery took over fourteen hours and they managed to get you through it, despite a lot of internal bleeding. Afterwards, you lingered between life and death for a few weeks. Dr. Tom told me to get your affairs in order. We really thought you were not going to survive. I started writing your eulogy in my head. Then, Dr. Tom had one more idea; to put your weak body on the ECMO, the life support machine."

Tears started rolling down my face. Pat saw my distress, saying, "I do not have to tell you all of this now. The important thing is you made it, and you are alive."

I nodded in agreement and slowly spelled out on the communication card, "You started writing my eulogy? Really?" Pat nodded and held my hand.

The rest of the story would come in bits and pieces, according to how much I could take in psychologically. This was a blessing. This is a caregiver tip that Pat now shares with the family members of cardiac patients whom we visit in the hospital. It is better for everyone to proceed with caution.

The next morning, Dr. Tom and Dr. Sam came into my room during their morning rounds to check on me. Dr. Sam playfully patted my arm and said in his thick New York accent, "Did you bring the bagels? I want mine." His sense of humor made even the most horrible aspects of treatment tolerable. Both men had become family to us by this time.

Dr. Tom picked up the story where Pat had left off. "You were probably the sickest patient we have ever had to treat." Somehow, this was not reassuring to me. He continued, "We fought with your insurance company and told them that if we did not put the LVAD in you were going to die."

Dr Sam interrupted excitedly and said, "Yes. And we won!"

Dr. Tom told me the intervention that saved my life was the ECMO machine. He explained what the ECMO machine was and what it did for my body. "ECMO stands for Extracorporeal Membrane Oxygenation," he said. "The ECMO machine is similar to the heart-lung bypass machine used in open-heart surgery. It pumps and oxygenates a patient's blood outside the body, allowing the heart and lungs to rest. It was really our last chance with you after your LVAD surgery. Fortunately, your body loved it, and it saved your life." Apparently the ECMO machine has also been used to help patients with COVID, bringing them back to life as well.

After a quick evaluation of my surgical site, the doctors seemed happy with my progress and left to continue their rounds. I sat alone in the hospital bed, stunned. While I was damn lucky to be alive, there was still a very long road ahead of me on my way to heart recovery. At the present moment, I could not walk, talk, or do anything to take care of myself. As a former "Type-A" control-freak personality, I realized at this moment that my life would need to change forever.

I lingered in the CICU for the next week. I kept trying to use my voice, but it was hopeless with the intubation. Like Patty Duke in the old Hellen Keller movie, I stabbed at the laminated card, desperate for friends and loved ones to understand what I was trying to communicate. I longed to have the invasive tube removed from my throat. Dr. Kellie, a young female CICU resident, would not approve the removal of the tube. "Her lungs are too weak. I do not want them to fail on us again," she said to Pat one evening. I had the horrible feeling of being objectified; I sat there while two people had a conversation about me and my care, unable to communicate with them or add my opinion. Pat jokingly refers to this period of time as "the blessed silence."

I looked at Pat after Dr. Kellie left and pointed to the card. I tapped out W-H-A-T H-A-P-P-E-N-E-D? on the card like a pecking chicken.

Pat let out a long sigh saying, "Well, 99 percent of your organs failed before you went through LVAD surgery. Your lung and kidney function were almost gone. Their function is returning, but they are not strong enough yet to work on their own, so you are going to have to stay intubated for a while."

"A while" turned out to be five more grueling weeks of the CICU and intubation. I started to think Dr. Kellie saw me as a lab rat. While she was pleasant, she rarely told me what was going on with my condition. Instead, she would enter my room, check my vitals, and slip out without updating me on my progress. This infuriated me. In an act of desperation, when I saw my favorite night nurse, Carol, I tapped out the sentence: P-L-E-A-S-E T-U-B-E O-U-T?

She said, "Oh, I don't know when, but I will ask."

I smiled and tapped again: T-H-A-N-K-S S-O-R-E H-U-R-T.

Nurse Carol replied, "I know honey. I am sorry. She just

wants to make sure your lungs are strong enough to function on their own."

After six weeks, I was still struggling to get enough air in my lungs on my own. Dr. Kellie asked a surgeon to come to my room and perform an inpatient tracheotomy to help improve my breathing capability since my lungs were so weak. A kind male surgeon arrived with some surgical tools by my bedside. He apologized as he sedated me, then made the incision in my throat.

"I know this is not what anyone wants, but it will help you to breathe better," he remarked.

Since I could not speak, I thought to myself, *What is another scar? My stomach already looks like a roadmap for the County of Los Angeles.*

A few days after the tracheotomy, the intubation tube was finally removed. After they extubated me, the pain in my throat finally subsided, although I still could not speak. I felt one tiny step closer to getting my normal life back.

My daughters visited me the day after my tubes had been removed. They surprised me by decorating the sterile room with heart and flower stickers. The ten dollars they spent at the 99-cent store cheered me up more than any expensive interior design job I had ever experienced in my life. It is astounding how the simplest small acts of kindness make the difference to a seriously ill patient.

The girls visited me the day after my tubes had been removed and I still could not speak. This worried me. The hospital's speech pathologist visited me and explained that my throat would need to heal before my speech would return. I could grunt, but that was about it. He told me that, most likely, my voice box had been damaged by the intubation, but it would not be permanent.

My daughters and husband joked about the funnier

moments they shared during my coma. My immediate and extended family consists of world-class pranksters. My husband had thought about asking one of my nurses if my youngest daughter Annie could "borrow" an infant from the maternity nursery two floors up and walk into my room on the day I woke up. They had planned to show me the baby and inform me that I had been asleep for years and was now a grandma. Luckily, the charge nurse would not allow that prank to happen!

Pat had also considered taking a Sharpie marker from the nearby nurse's station and having my older daughter Claire draw a large mustache on me. They schemed about putting a sombrero on my head and a guitar in my hands, then taking a few photos. As crazy as these ideas were, they helped my family to cope with the intensity of what was going on. I was happy to smile and share a few laughs with them, even if it was at my expense. I have noticed in visiting other heart patients that those who recover the quickest are those who keep their sense of humor fully intact. These funny shared times helped to offset our family's difficulties during my recovery. Our family counselor told both of my kids that it was important that they try to keep life as normal as possible, despite the fact that their mom was in the ICU for many months.

We had our share of the very serious moments, too. I am not sure how Pat dealt with them all, other than being superhuman. One well-meaning coworker decided to visit me while I was still in the medically induced coma. Pat warned her that I was hooked up to a lot of machines and looked more cyborg than human. Still, this coworker insisted on visiting me. She walked into the hospital room, took one look at me, and fell apart emotionally. My mom and daughters were also in the room, witnessing this uncontrollable breakdown. Pat quickly walked my distraught coworker out of the CICU. He spent another hour calming her down before she drove home. The man, in my opinion, is eligible for sainthood. He dealt with many groups of people coming and going to the CICU over my three months of residency there. As he tells it, some days were easier than others.

Pat was a favorite visitor to the CICU with the staff. His mom Dorothy had been a public health nurse for almost fifty years, so he knew that humor was essential during a health crisis. When I was in the medically induced coma, Pat would enter the CICU, announcing his arrival by saying, "Has anyone here seen my wife, Darla Van Winkle? She's been sleeping for a long time." Pat brought a sense of joy and relief to the staff who worked so very hard to save my life. It is a small wonder that he is my best friend and that we have been married for thirty-five great years.

People often ask me what helped me survive those long months I spent in the hospital and CICU. All joking aside, my Viking and Celtic heritage helped. I was not ready to go to Valhalla and was too stubborn to die. My family and my medical care team saved my life. Even when I was in a coma, I could still sense the love that surrounded me. There is an odd awareness that even someone in a propofol-induced state can sense. Not one tiny prayer or act of kindness given to me at this time was wasted.

One of the most amazing acts of kindness during this time was from my CICU night nurse, Marilyn. She was a shy, unassuming woman who did her job with love. After one particularly grueling day of medical tests and not-so-good news, she came into my room at 4:00 p.m. and said, "You look really sad tonight, Ms. Darla, what is going on?"

"Well, I did not get great medical news today about my heart. But do you know what is really bugging me? My hair," I replied.

She looked confused. "Your hair?"

"Yep. I cannot remember the last time I had it shampooed with real soap, and the caps they put on you with dry shampoo really do not do a lot. I feel like a troll," I murmured.

After some thoughtful consideration, Nurse Marilyn brushed my hair and discovered that it did stick to my skull. After sixty days in the CICU, the lack of fresh air, water, and other key elements for life was taking its toll on me physically and emotionally She leaned over my bed like an excited teenager and whispered, "I will tell you what. Tomorrow night I will come by your room and surprise you. I will help you feel better." I smiled. Marilyn really went beyond her job to help people who were hurting. "Okay, that would be great," I replied.

The next evening, Nurse Marilyn arrived right on time with a large duffle bag. "We are going to do a little *Steel Magnolias* routine in here tonight and get you done up right!" she quipped.

Just like Truvy in *Steel Magnolias*, she produced a large bowl, some real shampoo and conditioner, a towel, blow dryer, and curling iron.

"Has your husband been by yet today?" she asked.

"No, not yet." I responded.

She then proceeded to draw the curtains, sat me in the patient chair next to the sink, placed the large bowl in it filled with warm water, then laid my head back. I have always loved getting my hair done, but this was about more than superficial beauty. She treated me with loving care during the next hour, washing, drying, and curling my hair. It was a small act of kindness that showed so much compassion that I still cry about it to this day.

When my husband came into my room, he smiled saying, "There she is! My beautiful wife."

I am not a vain person. But somehow, the act of looking better helped me to have better scores in my medical tests the next day, too. Nurse Marilyn, through a simple act of giving her time and talent, had brought me into the realm of the living again. Her acts of kindness were more powerful than all of the drugs I had taken in the hospital. She is truly an extraordinary human, who I go to visit on a regular basis. I always make sure my hair and makeup look on point when I say hello. It is a little joke we share between the two of us. The world needs more people like Nurse Marilyn. Or should I say, Truvy from *Steel Magnolias*. That is my official nickname for Nurse Marilyn.

The next lesson I learned as a transplant patient is that along your healing journey, many people will offer you small acts of kindness. Accept them with gratitude. They can mean the difference between recovering from a long-term illness and not recovering. And good hair helps, too.

14

CARDIAC REHAB AND NURSE ARLENE, THE DRILL SARGENT

AFTER MY BREATHING became stronger and my speech returned, I was transferred to the regular cardiac floor, known as a "step down" floor. The room was nicer with big picture windows. It was a relief to get out of the stodgy CICU basement. I would be in the step down room for only a few days before being transferred to the cardiac rehabilitation unit at another Scripps facility in Encinitas, California. Once at this location, I would begin my cardiac rehab. It would consist of physical therapy and occupational therapy. I had no idea at the time how mentally and physically challenging this next phase of my recovery would be.

My next lesson as an LVAD patient would be that cardiac rehab was not for wimps. I needed to relearn everything about functioning in life, from brushing my teeth to putting on my shoes, while being tethered to the piece of million-dollar equipment that had saved my life. While I was grateful to be alive, I was very nervous about the road that lay ahead of me. "How in the heck am I going to shower with this thing?" I asked myself. I would soon find out.

One bright February morning in 2012, my nurse on the step down floor told me I would be getting transferred to the rehab facility immediately. Randomly, the Amy Winehouse song "Rehab" started playing in my head. I laughed to myself, thinking that my brain had been affected by the large doses of anesthesia I had undergone during surgery. I was transported via gurney and ambulance from the La Jolla hospital to the Encinitas rehabilitation hospital. It was the first time I had been outside for months. The rehab facility was the last hurdle I needed to clear before going home.

The move from Scripps Green Hospital in La Jolla to the Scripps Rehabilitation Hospital in Encinitas seemed like it required a flight plan. Two teams spent four hours getting me from one facility to the other via ambulance. My new LVAD came with its own remote kit. The ambulance staff made sure I was fully connected to my batteries before moving me on the gurney. The backup unit that would be at my home was as big as a coffee table and was also transported. I wondered if my future journeys from home would be this complicated. When we arrived at the facility, the receiving end staff were completely prepared. I was the thirteenth patient who had been implanted with an LVAD at the La Jolla facility. The team had become experienced in dealing with the complexities of transferring LVAD patients.

My new room was bright and airy. It was a definite upgrade from the ominous rooms in the main hospital. I had so many mixed emotions. While I was extremely grateful to be getting my strength back, I was daunted by the thought of all the new equipment now attached to my body. I also considered that I might need to live with my LVAD indefinitely if a transplant organ could not be found.

Within an hour of being admitted, there was a sharp knock on my hospital door. A perky, petite woman entered my room.

She smiled, saying, "Hello, my name is Arlene, and I will be your Nurse Drill Sargent." I laughed and bonded with her immediately. She was tiny but tough and told me she was proud of her black belt in martial arts. Arlene shared with me that she was Filipino. I joked by asking her, "So did you bring my favorite lumpia with you?" Once again, humor helped us both to navigate the patient-nurse relationship.

Nurse Arlene handed me a copy of my daily schedule. I was shocked. The day was highly structured with many activities. "Your lounging days are over," she quipped. "Tomorrow will start with breakfast at 6:00 a.m., dressing at 7:00 a.m., physical rehab from 8:00 to 10:00 a.m., then occupational therapy from 10:15 to noon. After a one-hour lunch break, the cycle will repeat itself, ending at 4:30 p.m."

I sighed so loudly a nurse waiting outside my room stuck her head in to make sure there was nothing wrong. Getting my sea legs back was going to be a full-time job.

As Nurse Arlene saw the uncomfortable look on my face she said, "I have only one rule. You may not feel sorry for yourself. You may get mad, and you may want to quit. You are going to have to learn to do things again that were easy for you to do as a child. I ask that you be patient with yourself and with us. I would rest up today. Tomorrow you are going to need your strength." She turned and left the room.

I was stunned. Cardiac rehab was no place for sissies. Perhaps there was a reason that Nurse Arlene held a black belt — to whip her patients into shape!

The next day began early at 5:30 a.m. with a visit from the site phlebotomist. A tiny Hispanic man entered the room and whispered, "Hi Darla, my name is Jose. I need to draw a sample of your blood. Is that okay?"

"Sure," I replied groggily and stuck out my arm. I watched

him pull out ten tubes, all in different colors. "Every color in the rainbow, eh?"

Jose smiled and replied, "Yes, you are correct. When we take all these tubes of blood, we call it a 'rainbow draw.'" I laughed. Perhaps I would pick up an honorary medical degree after so many days spent with the staff.

I saw Jose almost every day, and we became good friends. He confided in me that many of the older patients became angry when he came in to do their blood draws. He did an excellent job; I watched the needle go effortlessly into my arm as he did his work. Jose told me to always ask for a green butterfly needle when someone drew my blood. My veins were very tired and covered in scar tissue from all the surgeries. The green butterfly was a tiny needle that helped weak veins to cooperate.

After Jose left, my breakfast tray came in at 6:00 a.m. Brenda, the cafeteria worker, slid it on to my bed table, saying, "One cardiac diet special."

Honestly, the food was not so bad. I was happy to have someone else making my meals. Once in a while, my friends would occasionally bring me treats during their visits. A particularly good friend managed to smuggle in a few tacos, although I doubt they were "cardiac friendly."

Right on schedule, Nurse Arlene arrived to help me get dressed. Despite her tiny frame, she managed to help me get up and pull on my sweats and t-shirt, then handed me my socks and shoes. "You can't put these on yet, because of your incision," she said. "I'm going to leave that up to your occupational therapists when they arrive."

I am a proud person. The kind of person who does not like other people to do things for them, especially personal things. It took me a while to adjust to the therapists having to help me with the most mundane daily tasks — from tying my shoes to helping me go to the toilet. My two occupational therapists, Jeff and Lauren, were the best. They offered me dignity in some very embarrassing situations. They helped me get over my frustration at not being able to do things quickly or well. After my experience, I consider physical and occupational therapists to be superheroes for the patience and kindness they show to their patients.

The first job we tackled together was tying my Nike athletic shoes. I had done this so many times, but never with an LVAD attached. The machinery made it a logistical nightmare.

Jeff handed me a funny-looking reach device, saying, "The only way those things are going to get tied is if you use this." I used the device, and it helped me to grab the laces and pull them into an awkward knot. The entire effort for both shoes took twenty minutes.

Seeing my discouragement, Lauren said, "Don't worry, it will get easier, and you will improve." I looked at her with an expression on my face that read, *You have to be kidding me.* Putting on my socks and shoes had taken all of the time allotted for the occupational therapists. What used to take me five or ten minutes to do at home now took me an hour to complete with all of my LVAD equipment attached. I sat down in the wheelchair, exhausted. Nurse Arlene appeared with some orange juice. "You have this, girl. Just keep going and hang in there."

My next appointment was in the physical therapy gym. Nikki, my physical therapist, approached my wheelchair in the hallway and introduced herself. With her muscular build and Eastern European accent, she reminded me of a Russian gymnast. "Let's go make you strong!" she shouted with enthusiasm. She whisked me away in the wheelchair down to the gym. The next hour consisted of grueling stretches, squats, and walking. The exercises that used to be my morning warmup were now the main event.

After an hour of physical therapy, she returned me to my room around lunchtime. I sat in the chair and looked out at the beautifully manicured grounds. It was hard to believe that my body had forgotten forty-nine years of muscle programming. Cardiac rehab was my only road back to independence.

After a week, my occupational therapists focused on teaching me about my shower routine. With the electronic LVAD attached, I was terrified. I pictured myself getting shocked or electrocuted. Nurse Arlene arrived with the "care kit" issued by Thoratec Incorporated, the medical device company that built my LVAD. It was part of the million-dollar equipment.

She tried her best to buoy my depressed mood. "Look at all these fun things!" She took out a black rubber briefcase and removed what looked like a Duck Dynasty hunting vest.

"Don't tell me I have to wear that ugly thing," I said bitterly.

"If you want to move by yourself, you do," she replied unapologetically.

Although the vest was ugly, it was functional. It had two side pockets which held giant lithium batteries. She handed me the rubber briefcase and said, "Okay. Now walk to the shower." Feeling ridiculous, I joined the two occupational therapists in the small bathroom. I had worn my one-piece bathing suit to hold on to whatever shreds of dignity I had left.

Jeff told me to unbuckle the LVAD from my waist and hang the briefcase over my shoulder. I took it off for the first time since my surgery. I gingerly placed it inside the briefcase and fed the lead through the hole in the side closest to my abdomen. It took me twenty minutes to do this mock preparation for showering. Jeff then instructed me to walk into the shower. No one noticed that some water had spilled on the floor earlier that morning while I was brushing my teeth. It was just enough to make the floor slippery and caused me to fall directly on my butt, with the suitcase in hand.

This slip and fall must have been a common occurrence at the rehab hospital. Jeff and Lauren immediately went into triage mode. Jeff instructed Lauren to stay with me while he filed an incident report. The attending doctor came in to check my equipment and make sure everything was still connected and functioning. Arlene brought in the charge nurse who had to report the slip-and-fall accident for hospital records. I was defeated and embarrassed. I looked up at them with tears in my eyes. My frustrated brain sent a message loud and clear to me: *This is your new normal, Darla.*

This was a bad day for me. We all have them as patients. The incident triggered my depression about having to rely on other people to get well. I sulked in my room and did not touch my dinner tray that night. My friend, Jim, another transplant patient who had been through many of these events, came to visit me. Dr. Tom asked Jim to visit me in the rehab hospital and act as my mentor during my LVAD rehabilitation. He provided me with friendship, support, and the occasional kick in the butt I needed to stop feeling sorry for myself on the long and arduous road to recovery.

He brought me a frosty chocolate milkshake, handed it to me and said, "You've earned this, kid."

I quickly confided in Jim about my concerns with the physical therapy unit. "It's going to take an eternity for me to become independent enough to return home," I said in a forlorn tone. He was quick to snap me out of my pity party. "Think of all the people who worked so hard to save your life and get you here, Darla. You are one of the lucky ones who has survived the LVAD surgery. Many have not." Jim's honesty and directness helped me to realize that I had nothing to complain about. I use this same tough love technique when I visit patients in the hospital now.

The following day, I woke up and saw from the calendar that I had been at the rehab facility for two weeks. When Nurse Arlene delivered my breakfast that morning, I asked her how much longer I would need to stay. She had been asked this question by many patients and responded, "Okay. Let's do a countdown on your board. I will be right back." She disappeared to consult with the doctor on duty. He confirmed that I should be ready to go home in about two weeks, if I kept making good progress with my OT and PT sessions. This was just the news I needed to keep at it. Nurse Arlene knew how to motivate her patients.

She drew a series of fourteen boxes on the white hospital board in my room. This was a visual reminder of my schedule for the next two weeks until I got to go home. There would be fourteen more days of arduous physical and occupational therapy, but I was up to the challenge. I was getting very excited. It had been over three months since I had been home. It's funny the things that you miss when you are hospitalized: the drooly kisses from your dogs, the smell of freshly baked cookies, flowers from your yard. It was the simple things I missed the most.

During the last week, Pat and I were told that we would have to pass two LVAD tests prior to my discharge. The first was a written test on the LVAD manual, which was provided by the manufacturer in an effort to educate patients and reduce product liability. The second was a hands-on twelve-step physical dressing change that Pat would need to do three times a week once we got home. The phonebook-sized manual was clearly written by an engineer; it had complex diagrams and instructions that could have been used for rocket-building. The manual cover featured multiple photos of smiling grey-haired citizens as they shopped, read, and played golf with their LVADs. I was relieved that Pat, an accountant, was the one who had to master the technical aspects of living with the LVAD.

Somehow, we were supposed to digest all of the information in the 226-page manual and pass the multiple-choice test on the LVAD with one hundred test questions. We would need to score 95 percent or better on the test items or we would fail. No pressure. If we failed, we would have to wait a week before testing again. Despite the fact that Pat and I hold five graduate degrees between us, we were both very nervous. We read the manual and took the test, passing with 95 and 98 percent — Pat got the better score.

The second test was a practical exam. Pat, as my main care-giver, had to demonstrate in front of the medical staff that he could successfully complete the twelve-step sterile dressing change of the LVAD incision site. I do not think either one of us envisioned this level of "in sickness and in health" when we got married, but that is exactly what it was. Pat scrubbed up and started setting up the sterile field with the supplies. As he began the dressing change, I was overcome by his love and compassion for me. The laborious dressing change lasted forty minutes. He did an outstanding job and passed with flying colors. The LVAD coordinator laughed and asked him, "Would you like a job here?"

Finally, Nurse Arlene checked the last box on the white board, and we did a little celebration dance. It was my discharge day, and I was finally going home. The last few months had been tough but necessary. I learned how to cope with my long-term disease, heal the parts of my body that could be healed, and do simple daily tasks such as showering and dressing that I once took for granted. We packed up my things, and I was wheeled out to the car. A line of my health team personnel stood with flowers and balloons, applauding and cheering me on.

My new life with the LVAD was about to begin, without a safety net.

The next lesson I learned as a transplant patient is that occupational and physical therapy reacquaint you with your body after surgery, and that drill sergeant nurses are tough and full of love for their patients.

15

LIFE WITH THE LVAD AT HOME

AS WE TURNED the corner onto our street in my husband's truck, I had tears in my eyes. Many times during my long illness, I never thought I would see our home again. Now, almost four months after the hospital admission, I was returning. My kids made me a colorful "Welcome Home Mom" sign that hung on our front door. Our two Labradors had their own welcoming committee dance. My home looked foreign to me. I slowly made my way to a large chair in our bedroom and sat down, checking my LVAD settings. I was nervous about our ability to self-monitor this sensitive equipment which was keeping me alive without my medical team.

I looked around at the remains of my former life, starting with the chair I was sitting in. It was a giant recliner that had been my bed before I went to the hospital. It reminded me of the many nights I could not sleep unless I was sitting up due to the fluids that had accumulated in my chest. The road had been rough, but we had made it. I was so happy and relieved to have survived my near-death experience and to be back at home.

For the present I was wearing the black Duck Dynasty mesh vest. It held all the LVAD parts I needed to function. A home health crew would be by that evening to ensure that we had correctly hooked up the large generator unit that plugged into our bedroom wall. I wondered to myself if I would ever be able to move about independently again. This was a lot of expensive equipment to carry around with us. I constantly had to remind myself that this wondrous LVAD was saving my life and making my body stronger for transplant.

One day I decided to put a call in to the Thoratec people who manufactured my LVAD to thank them for creating this new life-saving device. I wanted to ask them who had designed their accessories kit with the Duck Dynasty vest, huge lithium batteries, and rubber suitcase for shower use. It certainly was not Coco Chanel. My call ended up with what is called a "patient communications expert." Having been the thirteenth person installed with the LVAD in La Jolla, it occurred to me that this was probably a new position. The patient communications expert was named Amy, and she was very kind.

When I asked her about the cumbersome accessories, she replied, "Yes, I know. People hate them. Honestly, they were sort of an afterthought as the development of the device was finished."

I responded, "Well, have you seen the size of the batteries? They are *huge* and heavy. Why isn't the technology better around them?"

Her voice dropped to a whisper, and she said, "Just between us, you know what it is going to take? It is going to take one of these engineers or doctors getting CHF and having to wear them as a user. Then they will develop smaller batteries and better technology. It is just too expensive to develop smaller units right now."

Next, we talked about the Duck Dynasty vest. "The men don't seem to mind it," she replied, "but the women hate it."

I asked her if a female version of the vest had been developed. She said it had not. My brain started to fire on all cylinders thinking of a fashionable alternative for women. I thanked her for her time and got off the phone. There had to be a better way to live with the LVAD in the world every day. I wanted to create a better holder for the device that would be easier and more fashionable to wear over the long haul.

The next day, my friend Maureen visited me. She was an expert seamstress and looked at the device as I sat on the edge of my bed in my sweats. I asked her, "Can you make something for me to carry this thing in public without dying of embarrassment?"

Maureen snapped into action and showed up the next day with her sewing kit. She measured my torso, the distance between the drive line in my abdomen and my arms, and shook her head affirmingly. "Yes, yes, I think we can work with this," she said, encouraging me. "What kind of fabric would you like it in?"

"Denim, because it goes with everything," I replied.

She said, "I will be back in a week with a prototype," and walked out the front door.

Maureen could make a designer dress from burlap. I was hopeful that she could help me by making a more attractive carrier for my LVAD. Perhaps we could even offer it to other female patients who were struggling like me.

True to her word, Maureen showed up a week later with the first LVAD backpack in a lovely dark chambray denim. We both squealed and laughed in delight when the leads to my LVAD fit through the holes and were able to hide the machinery. Once again, someone's love had saved the day. That night, after weeks of being sequestered in the house, Pat and I took

Maureen out to dinner to celebrate her success with camou-flaging my LVAD. She gave me a greater gift than a backpack — my dignity and the ability to feel like my old self again.

In the following weeks, I would check stores for messenger bags that could house my LVAD controller unit, batteries, and cords. While I loved Maureen's backpack, it would be nice to have a few dressier bags to take with me to meetings in public. Since I was not physically ready to return to work, I started volunteering with my doctors, visiting other patients who were diagnosed with CHF, and waiting for an LVAD implant. Many of the patients looked so hopeless and sad. It brought me great joy to show them that they could survive the surgery and be mobile again. The LVAD had improved my blood-pumping capacity quite a bit, and I was able to walk short distances during hospital patient visits without getting winded. Unfortu-nately, it did not help to improve my unpredictable arrythmias. I still feared that Sparky my defibrillator could launch anytime, anywhere. And it often did.

One day, I passed by the Tumi luggage store on the way to the hospital. I had always loved their bags. They were sleek, efficient, and good-looking. They were also very pricey. Dr. Tom had asked Pat and I to go to the Scripps Health Founda-tion Candlelight Ball. A denim backpack would not go well with the stunning ruby red dress I had selected for the event. Maureen had altered the dress with an opening to thread my drive line through. I saw a lovely messenger bag that looked to be about the same shade of red as my dress. I asked the Tumi salesclerk if I could try it and explained to him my situation. By some miracle, it worked! The bag had an opening where the drive line could go. The best part was the entire device could be placed in the bag out of sight. Despite the three hundred and fifty-dollar price-tag, I grabbed it. I was now ready for the Candlelight Ball.

The evening of the event, I got strangely nervous. It was the first public function where I would sit, eat dinner, and hopefully dance with my LVAD in tow. Dr. Tom and his wife Stephanie had asked us to sit at their table. I was back in social circulation and felt strong and empowered. Upon greeting us, Dr. Tom said, "You look absolutely beautiful." I beamed. He took a photo of Pat and I dancing, the LVAD between us. I still have that photo on my desk today.

The next lesson I learned as a transplant patient is that even the bleakest situations can be overcome with tenacity and love from others. Maureen's backpack and Dr. Tom's photo are evidence of that fact.

16

LVAD BARBIE

FOR THE NEXT FOURTEEN MONTHS, I took my LVAD everywhere with me. It was not as if I had a choice; it was connected to my body. I learned to shower with it and got over my fear of being electrocuted. I even interviewed for a job with it, since my old position had been given to another employee during my illness. I understood. During the four long months of my illness and coma, no one knew if I would live or die.

Dr. Tom took to calling me "LVAD Barbie" when he asked me to show up as a living LVAD model at his medical meetings. I thought the name was cute and actually embraced it. There was one conference talk we attended which was particularly memorable for me. It was a large cardiology conference for physicians and thoracic surgeons that took place on the West Coast. Dr. Tom had briefed me on what he wanted me to do. Pat and I sat in the front of the room, just like the other men and women attending the conference. Dr. Tom stood and began his lecture. He was fast becoming a national expert on LVAD implementation.

"Colleagues, I am going to present an interesting and

unique case to you," he said. "Let's say I have a forty-eight-year-old female patient who has been suffering with congestive heart failure since the age of thirty-nine. That is nine years to be exact. Let's also say that despite the use of medication, her AICD defibrillator/pacemaker unit, and everything else available, her heart is failing fast. What would you do?"

A dead silence fell over the room filled with cardiologists, until a young male physician in the back shouted out, "CALL A PRIEST?"

Everyone in the room laughed, including me, but we all knew what a serious situation this was. Dr. Tom continued: "Here is what we did. I teamed with Dr. Sam, our cardiothoracic surgeon, and we decided to implant her with the LVAD as soon as we could. By the time we could do the surgery, over 95 percent of her organs had failed."

After some oohs and ahhs, the cardiologists were curious. "Is she still alive?" one of them asked.

"How is she doing?" another one said.

Dr. Tom replied, "Why yes, she is doing just great. Would you like to see her?"

Feeling more like a PT Barnum side show freak than a patient, I slowly stood up and the cardiologists and surgeons cheered and applauded. I did feel like LVAD Barbie but was happy to be there to raise awareness within the medical community. I was younger than most of the LVAD patients, so Dr. Tom felt that I provided hope for doctors and their patients under fifty who wanted to live a full life. I helped Dr. Tom to show the other doctors that CHF hits all age groups, and that recovery is possible even in the toughest cases.

While I wore my LVAD, Dr. Sam and I appeared on a national Scripps Health commercial together and became living examples of what a doctor-patient team could do to save lives. It was a fun experience, even though the set make-up artist told me she had to make me "look sick" as she applied ugly beige lipstick to my lips. "We can't have you looking too healthy and vibrant," she quipped as she applied my makeup.

As of today, approximately fifty thousand people across the world have been implanted with LVADs. As the technology improves, that number will increase. I am proud to have been one of the early users and adopters in LVAD history.

The next lesson I learned as a transplant patient is that when one shares his or her experience, everyone wins. This includes the good, the bad, and the ugly aspects of treatment (with apologies to Clint Eastwood).

17

ACCEPTING TRANSPLANT AS A REALITY

ONCE LIFE with my LVAD began, Dr. Tom started having regular discussions with me about moving to transplant list status. This was a lot psychologically, although I was excited at the prospect of being transplanted. If I received the gift of an organ, I would be able to live without the LVAD and do common daily things I had missed like swimming. Still, I was troubled by what physicians call "survivor guilt" and the thought that someone would have to die to give me the gift of a new heart. Many people on the transplant waitlist grapple with survivor guilt even before they get transplanted.

It is important to remember that the reason I got an LVAD was to get my body strong enough to bridge to transplant. This meant that while the LVAD was keeping me alive, I was still very ill, and my heart could not function on its own. I started attending support groups for LVAD patients offered by Scripps Health. Any time I began to feel sorry for myself, I looked at the destination patients who could not qualify for transplants due to their age or medical conditions and would be joined to their LVADs forever. To stay positive, I reminded myself on a regular basis that I was very lucky being young enough to be listed for transplant. Most people over seventy are not considered eligible for transplant due to their age. Since I was in my late forties, I would also have a faster recovery and a better prognosis for healing without rejection of the organ.

My clinical visits to Dr. Tom also indicated that the electrical problems in my left ventricle were not improving. In fact, my Ejection Fraction had slipped again from nineteen to seventeen. Anything less than twelve required immediate hospitalization, and Dr. Tom began having earnest chats with me about the third treatment solution, an organic transplant. Another reason I loved Dr. Tom was his sheer honesty.

Dr. Tom leveled with me about the status of my condition. "The LVAD is keeping you alive, but your quality of life is not great. I want you to be able to swim again. I want you to have better mobility and to get your life back. The LVAD is a lifesaver but not the best solution in your case. A heart transplant is." I let the words sink in slowly. We were finally having "the talk" about transplant, after thirteen years of dealing with congestive heart failure.

During this conversation, my mind flashed back to the first evening when I received my CHF diagnosis and Nurse Peroxide said flatly, "You need to get on one of those lists. Do you know anybody?" No, of course not. Why would we know anyone? I thought ruefully. Now Dr. Tom was going to help me to know the right team to get me to transplant.

Dr. Tom advised me to call my insurance company and ask what our transplant surgery options were. As I drove home from his clinic, I thought to myself, *This is really happening. I am going to get listed for a heart transplant. From someone else's body*. It was a very surreal thought.

That evening, after Pat and I ate dinner with the girls, we talked. I told him about my visit with Dr. Tom and his recommendation to get listed for a heart transplant. It had been a long road. Pat's response was simple: "Whatever it takes, let's do it." We had no way of knowing at the time how much would be required of us to go through this process. We had just begun the road to heart transplant, knowing it would be a long and rocky journey. It was going to take the help of medical teams, insurance workers, clergy, family, and friends to get us through it.

During one memorable visit, Dr. Tom took my hands in his, looked me in the eyes and said, "I think we have done everything we can do here. It is time to start thinking about getting you listed for transplant." I agreed, and we discussed the next steps that would help determine the greatest chances of getting a healthy, transplanted heart.

The next lesson I learned as a transplant patient is that transplant is a journey, not an event. The patient may be the focal point, but it takes an entire tribe of people to get you there.

18

GETTING ON THE ROAD TO TRANSPLANT

IT MAY SOUND CRAZY, but my first step to getting on the transplant list was making a call to our insurance company, Aetna PPO. In all fairness, I must say that the folks at Aetna knew their stuff and were very resolute professionals. We were extremely fortunate to have good coverage. I do not know what we would have done without their support. Most likely, there would have been dire financial consequences from the cost of my multiple heart surgeries. Pat jokingly refers to me as "the four-million-dollar woman," as that is how much all of my cumulative heart surgeries have cost my insurance company to date. I was grateful that Pat had been at his company for almost thirty years and that he had very good insurance coverage.

Some of my other transplant friends were not as fortunate. My friend Cliff had to get emergency Covered California insurance when he was diagnosed with heart failure. He waited for eighteen months in the hospital for his donated heart. When he was finally transplanted, his body was so full of medication that he went into acidosis. This condition caused him to reject his new heart and he died. While his care team did everything they could, the hospital where he was admitted only did ten transplants per year compared to Cedars-Sinai's two hundred annually. As hard as it is to acknowledge this, sometimes one's survival comes down to the law of averages and insurance coverage. It can literally be a numbers game of odds.

My first call to the insurance company was surreal. By the time I had worked my way through the labyrinth of robot prompts, I was patched through to a "patient care representative." This woman told me that a transplant coverage request was beyond her pay grade (her words) and that a nurse coordinator would be contacting me within twenty-four hours. I hung up and made a list of questions to ask the nurse coordinator. I recommend that other patients write down their technical questions for insurance and medical providers, as it is easy to forget them when one is involved in highly emotional conversations.

Within an hour, a kind woman named Julie called me back from the company. I told her immediately that I was completely overwhelmed by the thought of transplantation and the costs involved. She replied, "Try not to worry. We are going to get you through this." I hoped she was right.

Next, Julie gave me information on where I would be listed. "We'd like you to go to a Center of Excellence for transplant. Now, where are you located?"

I told her we lived in San Diego and that my cardiac treatment team was there.

She sighed and said, "Your closest one is going to be Cedars-Sinai Hospital in Beverly Hills, Los Angeles."

There was a long pause, and I asked her if we would need to temporarily relocate from San Diego to Los Angeles for three months.

Julie replied, "Yes, I am afraid so. They do more transplants than anyone and have one of the best track records. We want to get you the best medical team we can. Living next to the transplant hospital for two to three months is one of our requirements." Later, I would realize that this requirement is to ensure that if there are complications, the patient will be close to where the transplant surgery occurred.

This information was a lot to take in. In order to get our medical bills covered, we would need to go through the Cedars-Sinai protocol in Los Angeles, get me listed, then live there after the transplant. This was assuming that we had no complications after the surgery, and that everything went well. My mind immediately went into coordination mode, trying to figure out how we could temporarily move our busy lives for a few months.

I thanked the transplant coordinator for her time and got her contact information. She had given me instructions to ask Dr. Tom to do a "write-up" for a referral for transplant to Cedars-Sinai Medical Center. Dr. Tom had done this for many patients and was eager to see me get listed. Within a week, Dr. Tom and his staff had written up the referral, explaining to the Cedars-Sinai team how my condition had been worsening despite the drug therapy, AICD, pacemaker, and LVAD installations. The last sentence of his referral report said, "Clearly, an organic transplant is the only thing that is going to save this young woman's life." Seeing this in writing, I realized how very sick I had actually become. I was very thankful that things were moving ahead, as my quality of life was still not great.

Over the next few months, we waited as my condition worsened and my ejection fraction continued to drop to a very weak fourteen. Two months after receiving the referral report, the transplant team at Cedars called Dr. Tom. They told him on the phone that I was an ideal candidate, except for my weight. My

CHF had destroyed my metabolism. I was unable to exercise, and some of my cardiac medications had caused substantial weight gain. Despite steady effort on my part and some resulting weight loss, I was still about sixty pounds away from an ideal body mass index (BMI) for the transplant. Dr. Tom and I continued to be frustrated. On one visit, when the scale would not move, I jokingly said to him, "You could just lock me up in a cave and starve me until I meet the weight requirement." He laughed.

Dr. Tom was at his wits' end and decided to take things in his own hands. He conferred with his friend, Dr. Bhoyrul, who performed gastric sleeve operations. After a lengthy discussion, they agreed that a gastric sleeve would be the quickest way to get me "transplant ready" and below the ideal BMI that Cedars wanted. I told them I would do anything to get to transplant status and agreed to the surgery. The procedure was done arthroscopically, with my LVAD attached to my body. I was the first patient ever to undergo this procedure with an LVAD attached. I was proud to test pilot this surgical solution for other CHF patients who faced this same predicament. Today, this gastric sleeve surgery has been successfully performed on hundreds of Dr. Tom's patients with their LVADs installed in order to get them ready for transplant and other cardiac procedures.

After the gastric sleeve, my body began to drop weight quickly. I was within nine pounds of a normal BMI for my age, but the Cedars Transplant team still required more weight loss. My heart was dangerously weak and having more arrhythmias every week. Dr. Tom finally had enough. He sent a team of his nurses and residents up to Cedars to appear before the transplant board to advocate for my case. My nurse practitioner Laura and two young cardiology residents drove up to L.A. on my behalf. They presented my case to the Cedars-Sinai transplant team, saying that without an imminent placement on the list I would die.

The transplant board responded favorably to their testimony and approved me to be listed as a "1A" or top priority transplant. The victory had finally been won, and I was approved to begin the transplant protocol at Cedars-Sinai. People will often ask me why it takes a team to get you to and through transplant. Based on this experience, I reply, "If your doctor will not advocate for you, then find another doctor. You will not get to transplant status by yourself."

After the transplant board at Cedars-Sinai approved me for their evaluation protocol, they scheduled me to join the next group that would be going through the process. It is interesting to note that hospitals consider groups of people at a time for transplant. There are so many of us waiting for transplant that it is the easiest way for their teams to determine who is the most eligible.

I called the Cedars-Sinai Heart Transplant Clinic and registered. While I was excited, it was a daunting process. Jenna, the transplant coordinator assigned to my case, told me she would be my main point of contact from the Cedars-Sinai team. Jenna was courteous but direct: "Make sure you get here on time. If you miss your protocol appointment, it will be difficult to get you another one."

I told her we would be there.

The morning of our protocol evaluation date came in early February of 2015. We left San Diego at 6:00 a.m. in order to arrive by 9:00 a.m. when the protocol began. We sat through three hours of southern California traffic, mostly in silence. Pat and I knew we were in for the ride of our lives and had run out of conversation. By the time we reached the Cedars-Sinai parking structure, we were relieved. We made our way into the building, walking past the large reception lounge. The silent elevator whooshed up us to the fourth floor where the Cardiac Transplant Center was situated. We had already made several visits to this Center when I was getting my pre-protocol testing.

Shortly after being admitted by the Transplant Clinic, we were ushered to a huge, wood-paneled conference room. Other families were entering with their loved ones, and we sat facing each other around a massive, circular table. I recognized one of the Cedars social workers who began handing out light blue binders with a serious-looking cover photo that said "ADULT HEART TRANSPLANT" on the cover. It was tabulated with various directions regarding the long day of protocol ahead of us. This binder would become our resource guide for the protocol process, transplant surgery, and recovery.

Dr. Ken, the head of the Transplant Unit, appeared at the podium to make opening remarks. He was a gentle Japanese man with a soft voice. He addressed us by saying, "Good morning. You have been referred for heart transplant evaluation because your doctor feels that transplantation may help you. The evaluation protocol will help our team to decide if a heart transplant is your best option. During the evaluation, you will meet many people, have blood tests, x-rays, and other procedures. These tests will help us to decide if transplantation would be beneficial to you. Sometimes we find something that would make transplantation too risky for you. This could be an infection somewhere in your body, high blood pressure in your lungs, cancer, or thickening of the arteries."

I started to feel nauseous listening to Dr. Ken.

He continued his speech. "People you will meet during your evaluation include the transplant surgeon, transplant cardiologist, transplant psychiatrist, transplant registered nurse, transplant registered dietician, transplant financial coordinator, and transplant licensed clinical social worker." It was becoming apparent to all of us in the room that only those in the best condition for transplant would be selected for the surgery. The process began to feel like a marathon race where only the most fit runners would cross the line to transplant surgery.

Dr. Ken continued his speech, "In addition, you may need to return more than once to be evaluated by a neurologist, nephrologist, pulmonologist, physical therapist, and/or other specialists. The transplant nurse will help guide you through the evaluation process and answer any questions you have. The information from the test results and from each team member will assist us in deciding if you are healthy enough for transplantation and if it is the best treatment for you."

This felt like my first day of cheerleading tryouts on steroids. The stress was palpable. I had failed to make the cheer squad in high school. Would the same thing happen for getting a transplant? Despite Dr. Ken's pleasant demeanor, the more he talked, the more my anxiety grew.

Dr. Ken ended his introduction with some thought-provoking comments. "The evaluation protocol allows you to meet our team and learn about transplantation. You will learn about life with a transplanted organ and decide if you wish to pursue transplantation surgery. If you are accepted for transplantation, the final decision is yours and yours alone. In order to do well after transplant, you must be very committed and follow the instructions we give you." This was the final lap in my race to reclaim my life, and it was up to me to cross the finish line. No pressure.

The next lesson I learned as a transplant patient is that transplant surgery is a marathon process with very high stakes. Some patients make it, while others do not.

19

LE TOUR DE TEST

THE FIRST STOP on my protocol evaluation schedule was at the clinic's blood draw laboratory. This was an easy way to get the day started. Other potential patients going through the protocol schedule were not so lucky. I heard a middle-aged man griping loudly, "Why in the hell do I have to start with the transplant psychiatrist?"

I wondered to myself: *Does he get points deducted from his score sheet for that attitude?* I marched into the lab with a smile on my face, determined to get the highest score possible to be declared transplant eligible. This protocol process began to feel like *The Hunger Games* to some extent; only the "most fit" patients would be deemed eligible for transplant. The department coordinator explained to us at the orientation that although twenty potential patients sat around the large meeting table, only about eight of us would be accepted as qualified patients into the Cedars Transplant Program. When it comes to transplant, *the odds may or may not be in your favor.* I was determined to do the best possible job I could during the protocol interviews to become one of the lucky eight patients selected to move forward with transplant. In reality, I had very little to do with my destiny. My lab results would determine this outcome.

At the lab, I was greeted by Luisa, the elderly phlebotomist, who gave me a warm smile and a firm handshake. She led me into the room saying, "Hi, honey. Come and sit down and tell me about yourself."

Some of the things she was testing my blood for included HIV 1 and HIV 2, hepatitis B, the hepatitis C antibody, and any hyper/hypo thyroids. If any of these illnesses showed up in my blood panel, they would keep me from being transplant eligible. After the blood draw — a rainbow draw on steroids — she asked me for a urine sample. This would check for irregular creatine, urine toxicology, and other "no go" issues for transplant eligibility. In all of my life, I had never prayed so hard for normal lab test results.

Luisa bid us farewell and touched my shoulder lightly. I turned around and she leaned close to me, whispering, "Don't you worry, honey. You are going to make it. I can tell." I smiled back at her and hoped her prediction was right.

The next stop in our schedule was the cardiology transplant unit. Although I had already met the team, I would now have one-on-one interviews with Dr. Michelle, the lead female cardiologist who helped Dr. Ken run the clinic, and Dr. Brad, one of the top cardio-thoracic surgeons. Dr. Michelle entered the private exam room where the escorting nurse had left us.

After reviewing my file on the computer monitor for several minutes, she asked me some basic questions. "Do you follow medical advice and take your medications as directed?" "Yes," I responded. "I have been on meds for the past thirteen years and follow instructions for dosing every day."

Dr. Michelle smiled, checked off a few more boxes on a form we were not allowed to see, and told us we would be visited next by Dr. Brad, the cardio-thoracic surgeon. I started to feel like some medical version of Ebenezer Scrooge being visited by the three ghosts.

My husband Pat and I waited in silence. A few minutes later, Dr. Brad appeared looking like Dr. McDreamy from the television show *Gray's Anatomy*. He was young, handsome, and incredibly smart. He shook our hands and started in with the formal questions. "So, Darla, your heart function is very low, we know this. How have you handled the difficulties of your heart surgeries so far?"

Although I thought this was a more appropriate question for the transplant psychiatrist, I replied with my best job interview response: "Well, I have had four heart surgeries since getting my diagnosis. I have endured an AICD/pacemaker implant, several lead changes on those devices, an LVAD with eight pounds of equipment, and a gastric sleeve procedure to get me here today. It is safe to say that with this track record, I am motivated to get to transplant and to do whatever it takes to make my new heart happy and healthy."

Dr. Brad gave me a wink and said, "That's a very compelling answer and a good indicator of how you would handle transplant." He made a few quick notes and asked, "Do you have any questions for me?"

I asked, "Will you be doing my surgery if I get selected?"

He informed us that there were actually several transplant surgeons who worked on rotation, and that whoever was on call when my organ became available would do the surgery. His demeanor was so gentle and kind that I hoped it would be him doing my transplant surgery.

The evaluation meetings continued for another two hours, in which I had more cardiac tests including an electrocardiogram (EKG) and echocardiogram (Echo). At noon, we reconvened with the other candidates and their families for an informal lunch in the large conference room. As I glanced around the room, I saw exhausted faces staring back at us. The patients and their families looked like they were being put through an endurance race — which, in a sense, it was.

As I chewed on the tuna sandwiches provided by the Cedars-Sinai cafeteria, I made some mental notes. There were twenty potential candidates in my cohort. According to my research, only about eight of us would be successfully transplanted. Not all of us would pass the protocol, and of those who did, only some of the remainder would have a suitable organ donor found for them.

My birth mom was an unmarried sixteen-year-old who put me up for adoption as an infant. Because of the adoption, I had no knowledge of the diseases that could be lurking in my genes. I hoped and prayed for the best. During lunch, one of the Cedars social workers talked about next steps. She told us to make sure to send all of our test results for dental, ophthalmology, mammography, and colonoscopy to our transplant coordinator. Trying to be compliant, I had already sent these test results to Jenna the coordinator the first time she requested them.

After lunch, we had five more exhausting hours of protocol evaluation appointments.

During the social evaluation, the social worker talked with us about our feelings regarding my illness and the possibility of surgery. She made sure we had family available to help us after the surgery, including medical regimens, trips to the clinic, and daily activities. She emphasized that the strict treatment plan could be very complicated and stressful for everyone. Somehow, most of the transplant candidates already sensed that this was the case.

Next was the in-depth psychiatric evaluation. The goal of the interview was to determine how Pat and I coped with stress in our family life. It was also to ensure that neither of us had any drug or alcohol addiction problems. The psychiatrist reassured us that she would help us to deal with the stresses of the waiting period and the transplant process. I thought to myself, *I have already been waiting for thirteen years for this opportunity. Shouldn't I be used to it by now?*

The next evaluation phase was with the staff dietician. This worried me, as I had struggled to meet the BMI for transplant eligibility, despite the gastric sleeve procedure I had done. The dietician spoke with us about food and nutrition, asking me some hard questions. She leaned over and peered at me through her bifocal glasses, saying, "I can see you have had a gastric sleeve. Is overeating an issue for you?"

I bit my lip and fought my urge to say, "Yes, isn't it for everyone?" Instead, I smiled demurely saying, "I have done my best to work on any overeating tendencies. I believe I have proven that I have self-control through my recent weight loss in preparing for transplant."

She nodded slowly as she took notes. At ninety-eight pounds soaking wet, I wondered if she had ever dealt with a weight problem during her entire life. I could not wait for the evaluation process to be over.

Our next stop on the grand tour was the financial evaluation. We entered the office of the financial advisor, who was a young man in his mid-thirties. He shook our hands saying, "I have reviewed your insurance coverage and have determined what your benefits are, including prescription drug coverage. The good news is you are mostly covered for your potential transplant surgery and any treatment and medication it will require."

Pat asked what he meant by the term "mostly."

He responded, "Well, there will be co-pays for the hospital, surgery, visits, and drugs, but those will be minimal."

We sighed with relief. It was the easiest appointment we had all day. For others, it had been the most difficult appointment of the day. Those patients who lacked insurance coverage learned that they would be responsible for all medical treatment payments, including the million-dollar transplant procedure. We met a young couple in the hallway. The wife was in tears. She said audibly, "I can't believe I have to choose between a lifesaving transplant and keeping our home." Cedars and most hospitals do offer some financial assistance to transplant patients, but the burden of paying medical bills and pre-authorization usually comes down to the patient and their family.

After our last appointment with the nephrologist (blood doctor), we were exhausted. It was 6:00 p.m. We were on psychological overload from having endured more than a full day of nonstop interviews and tests. We celebrated by grabbing McDonald's burgers on the way back to San Diego.

Pat looked at me and asked, "Would the dietician approve of the calories in this meal?"

I smiled and him, saying, "I do not care. We are done with the protocol, and we are celebrating." The truth is, I don't even like McDonalds. I was just being a rebel after enduring hours of being on my best behavior.

The next lesson I learned as a transplant patient is that potential recipients need to show the world that they have the mental and physical stamina to become living recipients. There are no exceptions.

20

THE WAITING IS THE HARDEST PART — GETTING LISTED FOR TRANSPLANT

I HAVE ALWAYS LOVED the Tom Petty song, "The Waiting." I never knew it would become a personal fight song for me as I waited to get on the transplant list. A week after we endured the protocol evaluation at Cedars, we received a letter from them advising us of the "Decision-Making Process." The letter contained an advisory to patients. It stated that after all my tests were done, my case would be discussed by the transplant team members at their Patient Selection Committee Meeting. The team would then decide if I was a good candidate for a transplant. The team would make this decision collectively base it on the information they collected during my evaluation.

The letter went into detail as to why I might be approved or denied for a heart transplant. I was relieved that my CHF was considered to be "severe" enough to help me qualify. I was also happy to learn that I did not have any other heart problems that could shorten my life or increase the risk of rejection such as other existing infections. I did not have severe diabetes, an inability to follow a strict treatment plan post-surgery or any other complications.

I was only fifty-one, and the cut-off age for transplant was seventy years old. I had Pat as an available caregiver and my mental function was stable. Despite several of my organs failing during my hospitalization, they had returned to 100-percent capacity. I was not an alcoholic or prior drug addict. After reading these requirements in the letter, I was hopeful that I would make a good transplant candidate.

The last paragraph of the letter explained that after going through the Cedars Sinai Transplant Team protocol, if I was selected as a potential transplant candidate, I would be notified by phone by my newly assigned Transplant Coordinator. I would then be notified by a mailed letter of my initial listing status with UNOS. UNOS was the organ brokerage group and stands for United Network for Organ Sharing. UNOS manages the national transplant list that is used by Cedars Sinai Hospital.

I slowly folded up the letter and looked at my husband. "This seems more difficult than getting into Club 33 at Disneyland," I scoffed. Club 33 is a Disneyland exclusive membership with a huge waitlist. People pay tens of thousands of dollars to join. Rather than giving me rides and restaurants though, the transplant membership would save my life.

Pat did not respond. While I knew we had done our best during the evaluation, the process was now out of our hands. Lucy, the social worker who had been our escort during the protocol process, told us we would hear one way or another within a month. Three weeks had passed since that time, and we had one week remaining to receive the news. We were used to the "hurry up and wait" effect brought on by dealing with heart disease. Years of anticipating my test results had left us with an ocean of experience. Still, it was frustrating. My condition continued to get worse, and even Dr. Tom could not hurry the process along.

The following week, our Transplant Coordinator Jenna called. I picked up immediately upon seeing the familiar area code of Cedars-Sinai.

"Hello, Dr. Calvet?" Jenna quipped. "I have good news for you. You have passed our evaluation and will be officially listed as a 1A patient at Cedars-Sinai starting today. We have thirty days to try to find an offer of an organ for you."

I am not sure I heard much after the words "passed our evaluation" as adrenaline began shooting through my veins. We did it. Pat and I had survived the protocol evaluation, and I would be listed for the next thirty days with Wait List Status 1A.

"Do you have any immediate questions?" Jenna asked.

"I have plenty, but I will read over the information and write them down," I replied, trying to sound as low-key as possible. "Thank you, Jenna."

I hung up my cell phone, and Pat and I jumped around the bedroom like a couple of drunken rabbits. We had been through so much. I felt like a death row inmate getting a last-minute pardon from the governor. The road to transplant had begun.

Being a PhD research nerd, I immediately went on the United Network for Organ Sharing (UNOS) website at www.unos.org. I wanted to be as informed as possible of the different waitlist statuses and how I compared to other patients. I quickly learned the following aspects about "being waitlisted."

Please note that these listing criteria were current when I was transplanted in 2015; they have changed since that time and may be found on the UNOS website.

- The UNOS waiting list operates 24 hours a day, 365 days a year. (Death never takes a holiday, so neither does UNOS).
- UNOS monitors every match to make sure it is in compliance with the laws. The limited supply of organs is distributed fairly and according to the condition of each patient on the list.
- Patients on the waitlist are grouped into one of four statuses: Status 1A and 1B, Status 2, and Status 7 (Do not ask. There is no logic to this numbering system.)

STATUS 1A

- Patients in the intensive care unit on life support and/or high-dose intravenous (IV) medications to help their heart function.
- Have a ventricular assist device (VAD) or other mechanical device to help their heart. Device-dependent patients are given thirty days of Status 1A time automatically. (Did I mention I suddenly loved my LVAD and AICD?)

STATUS 1B

- Have a support device implanted and have not been transplanted during their initial thirty-day period of Status 1A time.
- Are receiving continuous low-dose IV medications either at home or in the hospital.

STATUS 2

- Patients that do not meet the criteria for Status 1A or Status 1B.
- These patients are usually waiting at home for a donor heart and are taking oral heart failure medications.

STATUS 7

- Patients that are temporarily inactive on the heart transplant waiting list. An example of a Status 7 patient would be a patient who has an infection and cannot have transplant surgery until the infection has cleared.

Your status on the waiting list may change over time, depending on your health.

I quickly surmised after reading the UNOS data that there was good news and bad news. The good news was, I was in the top Status 1A classification and had the best opportunity for getting a heart. The bad news was, regardless of my status, I would only have thirty days at the top of the list. The other not-so-great news was I had Type O blood, the most common type found in humans, meaning that I would be in competition with more people who also had my blood type and were waiting for precious organs. A patient waiting for a transplant with a rarer blood type such as AB positive or negative typically has a shorter wait time on the list. It is simply the law of probability at work.

The following morning, Jenna called again to confirm my status on the waitlist as 1A. This was not really a surprise to me since I had an LVAD. It was February 7, 2015. Jenna never minced words. She ended the call saying, "You are listed as 1A priority today. You will have thirty days, after which your name will expire on the list." Yes, she used the word *expire*. "Then you will be dropped to Status 7 until your case can be re-evaluated."

Other transplant patients had told me that Status 7 was basically the transplant equivalent to the Island of Misfit Toys. Once you were there, it was hard to get re-listed. The message was loud and clear: I needed to be matched with a donor within thirty days, or I would linger indefinitely and probably not survive.

The first week passed quickly and uneventfully. We did receive a wrong number one evening on my cell phone at one in the morning. It was a drunk teenager on the other end of the phone saying, "I am sorry, man. I was trying to call my mom for a ride." We laughed nervously after that incident. But I still wished it had been Cedars Sinai calling.

I phoned Jenna the following morning and asked her if some patients had multi-listed at other facilities. Apparently, she had been asked this question many times before. She responded, "You are allowed to be on the waitlist at other trans-plant centers. This may increase your chances of getting a heart sooner. Other factors may determine if this is a good option for you. You should talk with a nurse coordinator if this is some-thing that you are interested in."

I did not want to rock the boat or appear disloyal to Cedars in any way, so I told her, "Thanks, I think I will just list with you for now." I felt like I was rushing a sorority again as I did in college — waiting to be accepted into an exclusive club by an invitation bid.

And so, the waiting started. The first week was easy breezy. Then, when the reality of the second week hit, I started counting down days. I had written a large red "12" on the calendar. Only eighteen precious days remained for Cedars to find me a match. Time was going fast, and my patience was dwindling. Looking for solace, I consulted my Cedars Sinai reference documents for help. The documents stated that waiting for a good heart could take years or weeks. They also explained that this can be a difficult time for patients, and that they would have normal reactions such as denial, fear, anxiety, and uncertainty. I found during this difficult time that attending support groups helped me to keep my spirits up.

Since Pat and I lived in San Diego, we sought out local heart transplant support groups. The closest one was run by the team at Sharp Hospital near our home. We felt like medical tourists. The Sharp community was very tight-knit with its doctors and patients. Each person there was assigned a transplant number and literally introduced themselves with it. For example, one woman introduced herself saying, "I am Robin, and I am number 422." While I found this endearing, I felt like an outsider. None of the patients I talked with had been transplanted at Cedars except for my buddy Jim, who was not in the support group. While the group was welcoming, we felt as if we somehow did not belong. Still, I appreciated their outreach and support to Pat and me at a time when we needed it most.

Since I was not working at the time, I cleaned and organized the house to keep myself busy. I grew fatigued very easily, and one day all I could do was empty the dishwasher. Still, I tried to keep my mind busy and stay occupied. I considered what I had read about waiting time from the hospital documents. The time needed for me to find a heart would depend on my blood type, my UNOS listing, how long I had been put on the transplant list, and the size of my sick heart. My doctors had told me to rest up and not to go anywhere on travel during the wait list period.

For the time being, all I could do was wait and hope for that life-saving phone call.

The next lesson I learned as a transplant patient is that Tom Petty was right; the waiting is the hardest part, especially when your name is on the heart transplant list.

21

DIVINE INTERVENTION

AS THE THIRTY days wore on, I kept tracking my time left on the transplant list on our wall calendar hanging in the kitchen. I was up to day twenty-seven. The red marker on the current date glared angrily at me, causing me more anxiety. I had three more days at the top of the 1A list. I placed several calls to UCLA and Keck (USC) Medical Center in case I "expired" on the thirtieth day. Friends and family members called me, trying to buoy my spirits. I had shut down to pretty much everyone except my immediate family. I knew how many people died waiting for organs, and the number was staggering. That evening, I dropped to my knees and prayed to God not to be one of them.

In a childlike way, I spoke my petition aloud. "God, if you are listening, you know my situation," I prayed. "I have lived with this wretched CHF for thirteen years, and I am so tired of being sick. If it is in your will, please find me a donor heart. If it is not, I accept it, but please try your best."

I turned around and saw my husband Pat standing in our bedroom doorway. There were tears running down his face.

This is a man who rarely cries. We both knew that my situation had become very dire, and that only a miracle would fix it.

At 6:03 the following morning, on March 6, 2015, I woke up to hear my phone ringing. I immediately recognized the area code and Jenna's number. I tried to remain calm.

"Good morning," I answered.

"Darla, this is Jenna at Cedars-Sinai. We have an offer of a heart for you," said the familiar voice on the other end of the line.

My adrenaline started to race.

Jenna said, "We need you to get here within four hours. Drive safely on the freeway and go directly to the hospital for admission. Remember, this may or may not be a dry run. We are all rooting for you and will see you soon."

Typically, it takes about three hours without traffic to get from San Diego to Los Angeles. I hung up the phone and sprang into action.

I walked quickly into our living room where Pat had been reading the morning paper. He was always an early riser, taking our Labradors out for their morning stroll around 5:30 a.m. I sat down next to him, took his hands in mine, and said, "We got the call. God has answered our prayers. Let's go." The team at Cedars had advised us to have a bag packed for when this happened. Pat and I were good to go. We grabbed the hospital bag and quickly left the house. As we opened the car doors, I turned to him and said, "And don't drive on two wheels like Fred Flintstone." We hadn't been in this much of a hurry since going into labor with my daughters.

Our kids were both living away from home — our youngest Annie was on a year-long student exchange to Berlin, Germany, and our eldest Claire was a senior at Northern Arizona University in Flagstaff. We had asked our good friends to care for our animals once we received "the call."

Before walking out the door, I had slipped the "just in case" letter I had written for Pat and the kids on his desk. Here is what it said:

"If you are reading this, I have gone home to be with God. Please do not be sad. Please know that Dad and I did everything we could to treat my CHF and that, for whatever reason, the transplant did not work out. I want you girls to live your lives to the fullest. I want you to take every opportunity life gives you and to be happy. Dad will always be here to take care of you. Thank you for all your love and support, and one day we will be together again. I love you, Mom."

Other patients ask me if I felt sad writing this letter. For me, it was more of a necessity. I wanted to say goodbye to our adult kids in case something went wrong. Every heart transplant patient has to decide how they want to wrap up their affairs. This was the only thing I did to say goodbye to them before my twelve-hour transplant surgery. I hoped that my kids would never have to read that letter. I tell other patients I visit who are waiting for surgery that they need to do what feels right for them. It is just that simple. When I returned home after my transplant, I said a prayer of thanks and threw the letter away, thanking God out loud that they never needed to open that envelope.

The car ride from San Diego to Los Angeles went smoothly, and we miraculously hit very little morning rush hour traffic. We pulled into the now familiar Cedars-Sinai parking lot at 9:45 a.m. on the dot. During the drive, we texted messages to our friends and loved ones, telling them that we had received the call and that we would keep them notified as to what came next.

Pat grabbed my packed bag and we proceeded to hospital admissions. I remember lovely aquariums with beautiful fluorescent tropical fish along the walls of the admissions area. I thought to myself, *Look at those cool fish. I am getting a heart transplant today,* as my mind raced. A few minutes later, the admitting staff member called us. She was very direct. "Okay, so you are going in for heart transplant surgery today. This is what will happen. You will be admitted, go to a hospital room, and wait for the organ procurement team to notify your surgeon. Once your surgeon is called, we will begin to prepare you for surgery. It probably will not be until later this afternoon." She wrapped a paper hospital identification band around my wrist and directed us to the pre-operative hospital floor.

As my admission into surgery was beginning, my donor's life was ending. His family had to make the difficult decision to remove him from life support. The procurement teams were beginning to make arrangements according to what organs were being removed and transplanted. Teams were coming from all over to collect the precious gifts of Alex's thirty-year-old body and bring them to waiting recipients in other states. Emotions were running high for both the donor family and the waiting recipient families. This is the essence of the gift of life through organ donation.

The next lesson I learned as a transplant patient is that the arduous and incredible journey of being listed for transplant is well worth the opportunity of beginning a newer and healthier life.

22

SAINT ALEX, THE GOOD

SEVERAL FLOORS below my room in the pre-surgery suite, my donor Alex was drawing his last breath on life support. Three days prior, he had been admitted to another hospital for routine TMJ jaw realignment surgery. It should have been a simple, straightforward operation. His wife Kristina was told by the medical team that she could drop him off at six in the morning and pick him up later that day at four in the afternoon after his procedure. Her intuition told her to stay at the hospital. Within a few hours, the supervising surgeon came out of the operating room with an exasperated look on his face and some horrible news for Kristina.

The surgeon told Kristina that Alex had begun bleeding on the brain during the procedure and that there was nothing they could do to help him. For the next few days, Kristina had to make some of the most agonizing and selfless decisions of her young thirty-year-old life. She and Alex had only been married for five years but had managed to travel around the world to many countries together. They enjoyed a wonderful, sweet life together during his short time on earth. Now she was facing becoming a young widow and having to decide what she needed to do to fulfill Alex's wishes for organ donation.

Alex's instructions on his DNR (Do Not Resuscitate-Advanced Directive) were to donate all of his organs in the case of brain death. Unfortunately, that situation was happening, and Despite Kristina's mind-numbing shock and grief, she had to spring into action immediately to ensure that Alex's organs would be procured and donated according to his final directive. I cannot imagine the painful series of decisions that she had to make within a very short period of time.

Organ donation is a type of well-choreographed ballet by the procurement teams. Jenna, our Transplant Coordinator, gave me an overarching view of the steps during this process. First, a patient with a brain injury is identified in the hospital by physicians and will have in-depth testing. If these tests show no chance of recovery, the local Organ Procurement Organization (OPO) will be called. The Procurement Coordinator, who is well trained in organ donation, will then meet with the family to talk about organ procurement. The Procurement Team will make sure the donor patient is in good condition otherwise for the donation. They also ensure that the organs go the right patients who are on the waiting list.

The Cedars Sinai local OPO is named One Legacy. Most transplant donors come from local and regional OPOs. My local OPO was the Southern California regional OPO, One Legacy. Most heart donors are those patients who have suffered a serious brain injury either from an accident or from a disease such as a stroke. Most of them are sixty years old or younger. Since there is a substantial wait list for donor hearts, sometimes hospitals will consider hearts that are compromised, such as former drug addicts. There is full disclosure by hospitals if this type of compromised heart is being offered to the recipient. This was not my situation, so I did not have to consider the potential side effects. I have known other heart transplant patients who did accept compromised hearts from donors who had addictions and other illnesses. They have all had good results from these transplanted organs.

While I was being prepped for heart transplant surgery, my donor's organs were being procured by the One Legacy organ brokerage team. The Procurement Coordinator from One Legacy came to examine Alex's organs as they were being procured to determine whether or not they were suitable for transplantation. Alex helped many people that afternoon, donating both his tissue and organs. Since his heart kept his body functioning, it would be the last organ removed from his body. Although I had been admitted for surgery at 10:30 that morning, the surgeon did not come and introduce himself until 3:30 p.m., one hour before the transplant surgery would begin.

My transplant surgeon turned out to be Dr. Antonio. I had met him on a prior visit to Cedars, and he was not one of my favorite doctors. He was very direct and spoke plainly with a thick Spanish accent. At my sickest point, he had told me that I might never get a transplant because my body had grown too weak. I found it highly ironic that now he would be doing my transplant surgery after the LVAD had made my body stronger. I secretly wished that Dr. McDreamy had been my surgeon instead of this assertive dynamo, Dr. Antonio.

Dr. Antonio did not remember me from that prior visit when I was extremely ill. He walked to the edge of my hospital bed, made a tiny bow, and said, "We are going to do this heart transplant surgery now. The heart looks good, and I am ready to transplant it. We will start in one hour. I am going to scrub in." With those words, he turned on his expensive Bally crocodile-shoed heels and exited the room. Charm was not Dr. Antonio's strong suit. I whipped out my cell phone and Googled him. He was one of the leading transplant doctors in the world. I suddenly lost all interest in his personality. We were not going on a date; he was the surgeon who was going to give me a second chance in life. I thanked God for Dr. Antonio's expertise, and a surgical nurse came in to start the sedation medication in my IV drip.

Honestly, I do not remember a lot from those final moments as they wheeled me down to the surgical suite. People often ask me if I thought of my husband, kids, or extended family. I had come to a place of acceptance with the surgery. I was so grateful that a healthy heart had been found for me that I was at peace. The drugs probably helped too. Pat gave me a final hug and kiss, and we made our way to the operating room. Pat pushed my gurney until we got to the giant galvanized doors. I offered a quick prayer up to heaven that if I survived this surgery, I would dedicate my life's work to helping other transplant patients. Dr. Elizabeth Kubler-Ross, the social psychologist, calls this type of behavior "bargaining." I have kept that promise by visiting many patients and their spouses in the hospital who are waiting for transplant and writing this book to share my story.

Was I nervous before this monumental surgery? Not really. I had come to accept that I was given an incredible opportunity to begin a new, healthier life. My quality of life had become so poor — between the devices, medications and LVAD — that I was ready to face whatever was in front of me. Several of my heart buddies had told me that transplant surgery was actually easier than the LVAD surgery. I suppose you could say I reached a place of peaceful understanding before I went into the operating room.

Since I cannot see a thing without glasses or contacts, I only vaguely remember seeing rows of scissors, scalpels and surgical instruments on tables lining the walls of the operating room. I thanked God that I could not see very well. I probably would

have fainted if I had seen the equipment needed for the operation. I had started to fade before the anesthesiologist even asked
me to start counting backwards, and then, total blackness.

*The next lesson I learned as a transplant patient is: Relax,
God's in charge.*

23

THE LAMBORGHINI IN MY CHEST

I AWOKE the following day on the morning of March 7, 2015. It was Pat's fifty-third birthday and my new transplant birthday. Transplant patients often say that they have two birthdays — their original one and their second one on the day they are transplanted. I was confused for the first ten minutes. I looked around my hospital room, then felt down by my abdomen to see if my LVAD was gone. It was! The transplant surgery had happened, and it was a success. A wave of euphoria washed over me as I realized that the eight pounds of LVAD equipment had been removed from my body. After fourteen months of wearing it, I was no longer tethered to a machine. Best of all, I felt the warmth of blood circulating through me at full speed. This was the first indication that I had a healthy heart beating in my chest; my blood was flowing regularly for the first time in fourteen years!

A young male nurse entered my room who looked more like a linebacker than a Cardiac Intensive Care Unit staff member. "Ah, you are awake. Let's check your leads and see how you are doing with that new heart, okay?"

Once again, I had been intubated, in case my lungs were too weak to function on their own. I nodded in agreement and hoped that I would not be intubated for very long. It is extremely uncomfortable having a plastic tube jammed down your windpipe. I feared losing my voice again in the process, too.

The male nurse went out to fetch one of the cardiac senior nurses. Walking in, she said, "Wow! You are up already. It is only 6:30 a.m. and your surgery ended at 4:30 a.m. That is quite an impressive speed record," she quipped.

I smiled with relief — on the inside.

The nurse handed me a pen and a pad of paper and said, "Use this to write down what you want to know."

I crudely scribbled the words, "HUSBAND — PAT?" on the pad.

The senior nurse deciphered my scribbled writing and said, "Oh yes, we will call him immediately and let him know you are awake." Little did I know that Pat and his sister, the faithful Dr. Helene, had spent all night in the CICU waiting room and left the hospital at 4:30 a.m. that morning, exhausted. It had been only two hours since the time they left to go home when the lead nurse called him to tell him I was awake.

The nurse came back into my room, checked my vitals, and said, "He will be here as soon as he can shower and drive up. It will probably be about two hours."

I nodded in agreement that I understood. The next thing I scribbled was, "TUBE — OUT SOON?"

She responded, "As soon as the surgeon comes in and clears you. I know it is uncomfortable."

The fog of the anesthesia still lingered in my body. My limbs felt heavy. I closed my eyes and dozed, with the relief of knowing that my years of struggling with my ailing heart were over and I could begin a new path to recovery with my donor's strong heart beating steadily in my chest. At that time, I did not know anything about Alex's identity. I would not meet his widow and family until a year later.

Pat arrived within an hour. He looked exhausted but happy. It had been a long and bloody ordeal together, from the time I received the diagnosis of CHF until now, and I would not have survived it without him. I tell people that I fell in love with my husband all over again during this struggle. A lesser man never would have made it, and for that I will always be grateful. He beamed when he entered my room, smiling and kissing me on the cheek.

The charge nurse told him to be careful since I had so many leads attached to my body.

He looked at me smiling and said, "This is nothing; we've been through much worse."

Later that afternoon, Dr. Antonio came by to check on me. "Hello," he announced as he walked in my hospital room and clicked his heels together. "I put a Lamborghini in your chest last night," he said.

I looked at him, confused. I did not understand his car metaphor and thick accent.

"I put the best heart in your chest we could have wished for," he continued. "The donor was young, and he had an extremely healthy heart. You should be in very good shape for a long time if you take care of it. I was in there with you for a long time — twelve and one-half hours, to be exact. I am very happy with the results. Congratulations."

I looked at Pat in disbelief as he nodded, confirming this fact. Dr. Antonio then left to visit another patient, and I never saw him again.

Two days later, my tube was removed. I could speak in a whisper, eat broth, and clear foods.

I asked one of the nurses why the donor's heart sounded so loud thumping in my chest.

Mary, the veteran nurse on duty, said, "Oh, honey. You are so used to being sick that you do not know what a healthy heart sounds like. Your new heart is strong and beating like a drum."

At the time, I did not realize that I had a male donor heart. All I knew was that Alex's family had made their selfless decision to donate his organs the night before my surgery.

The next few days consisted of doing "laps" around the CICU (Cardiac Intensive Care Unit) floor. This exercise routine began the day I woke up from transplant. The nurses and doctors wanted me up and on my feet as soon as possible so that I could get stronger and recover faster. With my background as a competitive swimmer, I was happy to cooperate. By day four, I was doing ten laps around the floor on my own, without a cane or walker. I wanted to shout aloud how great I felt. It was unbelievable. I had been given a miraculous second chance at life.

The afternoon of day five, a technician came in to do an ultrasound echocardiogram of my new heart. Out of curiosity, I asked the attending physician, "Can I look at my old heart? I have read that some hospitals let patients hold their own heart in their hands after transplant."

He replied, "No, we do not do that here. As soon as your heart was removed, it was sent to the pathology department for analysis."

I found it interesting that each hospital has their protocol pertaining to this request. I had seen pictures of heart transplant patients on Facebook, holding their old, enlarged hearts in their hands while beaming after transplant. There would be no photo op for me. Part of me was relieved. My poor old heart had grown twice its size during my congestive heart failure, pushing other organs against my ribcage due to its massive size. I was fairly sure I did not want to see it in its monstrous state.

After I was hooked up to the echocardiogram machine, Pat and I peered in amazement at Alex's strong heart beating in my chest. After seeing so many images of my sick heart struggling to stay alive, the sight of it made my eyes tear up.

I also experienced my first small dose of survivor guilt. It is hard to accept that someone had to die after making the altruistic decision to donate their organs so that I might live. Even without information on my donor Alex, it was still mind-blowing to think about having someone else's healthy functioning heart in my body.

My transplant friend Jim and I made a bet before I got "the call." We had a healthy competition going. Jim told me that his surgery at Cedars was so successful that it took him only seven days to get released from Cedars Sinai to his Los Angeles apartment. Feeling competitive, I told him that I would beat his record and be discharged in six days. He laughed when I called him on the sixth day after my transplant, March 13th, and told him, "You owe me lunch. I am being discharged on day six."

Jim replied, "Nothing would make me happier than to sit down and treat you to lunch when you get back home."

On the day of my discharge, we had one final round of visitors in my step down hospital room: Dr. Claudia, the head pharmacist at Cedars-Sinai, her assistant, and our transplant social worker, Lucy. Dr. Claudia was a tiny Asian woman with a soft voice. She tip-toed into my hospital room with a large tote bag in her hand.

I joked saying, "Is that a parting gift for me?"

Not missing a beat, Dr. Claudia responded, "Oh yes. A very important one." She set the large canvas tote bag on my bed and said, "These are your heart medications."

I peered into the bag and saw over eighty pill bottles, a large binder, a blood glucose testing kit, and diabetes syringes. This would be my new normal as a heart transplant patient, but it was a small price for having a second chance at life. I tried my best not to be overwhelmed at the thought of taking more than eighty medications a day during my first phase of heart transplant recovery.

Dr. Claudia spent the next two hours walking us through our new medication regimen. I refer to "us" because my husband was the one running the show. Remember how Cedars grilled us about our collective ability to function as a couple throughout the transplant? Over the next three months, Pat would be required to take my blood every few hours, administer these medications, and provide insulin injections. Diabetes can occur as a result of transplant, and the pharmacist had prescribed insulin as a precautionary measure. Pat said it was no big deal after the LVAD dressing changes. I was so grateful that he was willing to take on this daily responsibility. I had staples running down the length of my sternum and was in no condition to be doing this post-operative care myself.

Before I could be discharged, Pat and I had to write out what my regimen would be. He took copious notes, and the new schedule looked as complicated as an FAA flight plan. Medications and dosages were listed, insulin and blood checks were scheduled throughout the day, and clinical visits were listed every day for the first two weeks. This would be our new job: taking care of the precious gift of Alex's donated heart.

We consulted the Cedars Sinai handbook to see what was ahead next in our transplant journey. It informed us that I would have multiple biopsies to check the condition of my new heart before leaving the hospital. It informed me that I would need to know and understand all of my medications and why I needed to take them. It also emphasized the need for me to be compliant with taking all of my medications to avoid going into rejection of my new heart.

We could always count on the blue book to tell us what time it really was. We had a strange love/hate feeling about it. It reminded me of one of those friends who will tell you truthfully when the new dress you bought makes you look fat.

Lucy, the cardiac social worker, had known us since we had showed up for the transplant evaluation. She had tears in her eyes when she walked us to the exit of the facility. "Now, you have your apartment set up. If you need anything, please call me. Even if it is groceries."

I cannot say enough about how personally committed the Cedars-Sinai staff were to us. Lucy stayed with me as Pat went to get our car outside of the admissions area.

"I can't believe we made it," I said to Lucy.

"Yes, you have," she replied. "But remember, the journey continues. Transplant is a process, not a single event. It is up to you now to follow our directions and get well."

As we exited the hospital Pat quipped, "The best birthday gift you could give to me is to never return here again for surgery."

I nodded my head in agreement. We walked out of the front doors of Cedars-Sinai and hoped for the best.

The next stop was the corporate apartment Lucy had secured for us before transplant. It was located above the Hollywood movie studios in Toluca Hills, Los Angeles.

I jokingly said to Pat, "Hey, maybe we could go tour the Warner Bros. lot or go to see a taping of *The Ellen DeGeneres Show*."

He smiled, but both of us knew I would not be going anywhere but Cedars for the next two months. The risk of infection was too great. The first chore we faced at the apartment was a blood glucose test, insulin injection, and a round of medications. I started to understand why the rigors of the evaluation had been so complex. Not even my horrible gag reflex was going to keep me from taking my eighty-plus medications per day. Pat became an expert in grinding and cutting them and hiding them in my food. Such is the life of a new transplant patient.

The next lesson I learned as a transplant patient is that the road to recovery is long and requires strict adherence to taking one's medications and following directions. You have pledged to take the very best care of your donor's heart as you can.

24

I LOVE L.A.?

PRIOR TO THE TRANSPLANT, Pat and I signed a written agreement that if I received a heart at Cedars, we would live there for three months after my surgery. This is required by many insurance companies to ensure that if problems arise, the transplant patient will be close to his or her surgical center. Often, it knocks potential transplant patients out of consideration for eligibility due to the costs involved. One of my transplant friends "Ava" has started a foundation called "Ava's Heart," which raises funds in Los Angeles to help these patients afford pre- and post-transplant housing.

We were lucky that both of our kids no longer lived at home and our animals were being taken care of by friends and neighbors. We were also very fortunate about Pat's work situation. He had worked at the same defense contractor as a corporate accountant for over twenty-five years. They allowed him to work virtually in Los Angeles for the first month of my recovery. We knew that we were very lucky to have this arrangement with his company. His co-workers were amazing with our family: They presented us with two thousand dollars in food gift cards that we could use in L.A. and once we returned to our normal life in San Diego. We felt very loved and supported, which was so important during the transplant process.

Still, Pat and I faced some challenges with our new temporary living situation. After living in a large home in San Diego for ten years, I quickly got cabin fever in the five hundred-square-foot corporate apartment. I caught up on my reading and taught myself how to knit by watching YouTube videos. Friends and family drove to Los Angeles to visit. My appointments at the Cedars Transplant Clinic were fairly uneventful, and my recovery was going well. I just missed the daily hustle and bustle of outside life. Pat would humor me by walking me around the complex like an old grandmother. I was not allowed to go out in public with crowds for the first two months. I was also told that wearing a face mask in public would become a regular requirement for me after my transplant due to my immune suppression. This was a transplant requirement even before the Covid-19 crisis hit.

About two weeks into my recovery, I decided to write to my donor family. I felt so compelled to thank them for this second chance at life and could not wait to write to them. I did feel some weirdness about living because of Alex's generous gift. I began experiencing the survivor guilt I heard about from other recipients. I realized I was alive because of his passing and decision to donate. I decided to check with the Cedars-Sinai handbook again for guidance. The handbook mentioned that to protect my donor's privacy, the only information that could be shared with the recipient was the donor's age and gender. Each OPO sets forth the guidelines on how recipients can contact donor families, so I decided to call One Legacy for its guidelines.

True to their word, the Cedars team did tell me that my donor was a thirty-year-old male. I picked out a beautiful card, sat down, and wrote a two-page note. It basically thanked Alex's family for saving my life in the most straightforward way possible. I told them about my family, my career, and what I hoped to do as a patient advocate after my transplant. I tried to think about what I would like to read if I had been in their position. It took me several days to decide on a final draft letter. It was a surreal experience, thanking someone for a second chance at life.

Sometimes other patients waiting for transplant will ask me about writing to their donor family. This is a highly charged emotional experience. There can be several outcomes and not all of them are pleasant. Some recipients never hear back from their donor families. The grief can just be too great. Others wait five, ten or twenty years before responding to the recipient. The best thing a transplant survivor can do in this situation is to treat the donor letter as a thank you letter and then let it go. For me, it was a cathartic activity that helped me to deal with my survivor guilt. Everyone and every transplant patient are different. I tell other patients to follow their gut and act accordingly. Recipients also need to realize that the donor family may want to connect with them, and this can continue the tenuous relationship between the two of them. I did meet my donor family eventually, but it is not always a happy situation. Even in my case, I would call it melancholy at best. Seeing the faces of Alex's family when they listened to the heartbeat in my chest was a miraculous but highly somber experience.

At Cedars Sinai, the UNOS organ brokerage serves as the sole connection between the recipient and the donor. Their staff offers guidelines for sending recipient-donor thank you letters. They recommend being honest and sincere. They also suggest leaving out specific religious beliefs that may conflict with the donor family's wishes. They provide advance notice that they will edit all letters sent between recipients and their donor families, eliminating any text that could cause distress to either party. I was not used to someone reading and editing my letters; it felt invasive, but I understood the logic and the need to protect both parties.

I would not hear from my donor's widow for almost a year, which was understandable. My letter was originally mailed to the family in April of 2015. Kristina replied in January of 2016. It was the best holiday gift our family ever received. We opened it the day it was delivered from UNOS and cried.

Jumping ahead three years, we hoped one day we would meet Alex's family in person. In 2018, at the American Heart Association's Heart Walk in Balboa Park, San Diego, we did just that. I met his mom, dad, four siblings, Kristina, and her new husband. Meeting Alex's family was a highly charged emotional event. If I had to do it again, I would choose a more private place to meet the family.

The meeting was bittersweet for all of us. We walked the five-mile race in Alex's honor. His parents told me that before his death, he was accepted into the UCLA program to earn his doctorate in education. I also hold a PhD in Education and they felt that Alex's dream would be carried out through the work I was doing in my professional life as university administrator. I wept several times during the walk. We had planned to go to breakfast afterward, but everyone was so mentally and physically exhausted, we decided to take a rain check. I am glad we brought our dogs; they provided some funny moments to break the tension. Our yellow Labrador Hailey was so hot during the walk that she laid down on a pile of ice one of the vendors had tossed in the grass. Alex's dad said, "Now that is one hot dog." We all laughed, having a much-needed moment of levity.

Our three-month stay in Los Angeles had many funny moments. I remember an incident on a sunny afternoon in

April of 2015 when we were driving back from an appointment at Cedars. The traffic was unusually heavy, even for Los Angeles. As we edged by Sunset Boulevard, I saw long rows of dark limos and flashes of photography. It was the annual Oscars Ceremony! I tried in vain to spot a celebrity, but before I knew it, we were winding our way up toward the Hollywood Bowl toward our apartment. We did feel somewhat isolated in those first two months. There was little to do but stick to our routine and hope that my medical appointments went well — which they did.

After a month of seclusion, I was given permission to take little outings to get groceries or walk in the park. I had to wear my mask at all times. Even a small trip to Trader Joe's market for groceries was a miraculous outing for me, getting out of the tiny apartment. I longed so much for normalcy that every plant and food item was fascinating. I laughed aloud when a young clerk walked up next to me saying, "Yes, aren't those heirloom tomatoes just GLORIOUS?" He did not know how much I missed my homemade caprese salad while I was dining on low-sodium hospital food.

At the six-week mark after transplant surgery, my medical team gave me permission to do longer outings while wearing my mask. We took our first official "field trip" to the Getty Museum for a few hours of art appreciation and beauty. It still holds a special place in my new heart. After fourteen years of dealing with congestive heart failure, I could finally walk up the stairs again to the museum without being breathless.

I looked at Pat with tears in my eyes saying, "I can't believe what a miracle it is to walk on my own again!" He took a photo of us in front of a Gauguin statue, and we sent it to our medical teams. It showed how truly happy and relieved we were that everything was going well.

Toward the end of the second month (May 2015), Pat had

some year-end accounting work that had to be done in the office. We scrambled to have family members fill in at the L.A. apartment while he returned home to San Diego. This was a very difficult situation for us.

The first family member who tried to help us thought she was on an all-expenses paid vacation in Los Angeles. She refused to take my blood or administer my insulin shots and left all day for the beach or pool. With a relative like this, who needs enemies?

Next, we invited a younger family member to come help us out. She showed up with a friend. Both were in their early twenties. During one weekend, they spent both nights in bars and clubs and worried me sick. This led me to the conclusion that care-giving is not for wimps. I started to appreciate what excellent care Pat had taken of me during the months of my illness and recovery. In an act of pure desperation, we called one of my older relatives who lived in Newport Beach, California, and asked for help. Her home was within the required fifty-mile radius of Cedars-Sinai and my transplant team. This meant that we could finally leave the apartment as long as we stayed within that fifty-mile radius. While it was not an ideal situation, it was a step in the right direction.

After commuting from Newport Beach to Los Angeles during the end of the second month, we asked for permission from our transplant team to move back home early to San Diego. My first heart biopsy showed that I was doing very well with no rejection. The Cedars-Sinai team had approved the cardiologist who would be following me post-transplant and granted us permission to return home after two and a half months. I was overjoyed. I missed the little things in my own home, like our two dogs and two cats. We drove home to San Diego on April 30, 2019. I had not been home since the morning we got the call.

The next lesson I learned as a transplant patient is that not everyone makes a good caregiver, no matter how much they say they want to help. A good caregiver is someone who does what needs to happen without question or a lapse in judgment. It is a difficult role to fill, and wimps need not apply.

25

HOME ON THE RANGE

THE JOY of returning to my own home and bed was incredible. Ironically, hospitals are a terrible place to rest and recover. If you are unlucky enough to be next to the nurse's station, you begin to feel as if you are on a bed in the middle of the runway at the airport. Sleep is almost impossible. It was a tremendous relief to return to the solace of our home once again.

What I did not anticipate before returning home was the horrible insomnia that affects most transplant patients post-surgery. When I asked my team why this happens, they replied that the body has incredible muscle memory, and goes into fight or flight mode after experiencing surgery. Most transplant patients are put on medications for sleep such as Trazadone to help us sleep each night.

The handbook from Cedars Sinai described insomnia as one of the predictable side effects after the transplant surgery. Other side effects mentioned included strange dreams, nightmares, and hallucinations. Being newly transplanted, I could also experience pain, discomfort, nausea and poor appetite, difficulty concentrating, weakness and dizziness.

Sleep is very difficult for most cardiac patients in the hospital. While at Scripps, I had been given Ambien™ to help me sleep. The drug caused me to hallucinate, and I dreamt I was in the Civil War, being tied up by confederate army men. As funny as this sounds, the dream and hallucination seemed very real. I started to rip out my IVs. A tiny ICU nurse leapt on top of me shouting, "No! Please stop doing this! You cannot rip your leads out!"

End of the story: no more Ambien for me. Before I was discharged, the staff psychiatrist had recommended Trazadone to help me sleep. Although I do not like taking sleep aids, I realized that I needed them. Luckily, Trazadone is non-addictive. I still take it to this day, or I do not sleep. The staff psychiatrist also put me on an antidepressant after my transplant, which troubled me. "Why do I need to be on this drug?" I asked. He patted my hand, saying, "Transplantation is one of the most stressful things that humans endure. You are going to need some help getting through the peaks and valleys of recovery." I did not like someone making this decision for me, but soon realized that everything in my life had changed and that the medication would help me through those transitions. Almost a year later, I did take myself off of the antidepressant and have not taken it since. It is a personal choice and up to the patient and how they are feeling.

Pat set up a "mini pharmacy" on my nightstand, with my corresponding pill schedule. Around the third month, my new post-transplant cardiologist in San Diego, Dr. Brian, told me I did not have any risk for diabetes and could go off of the daily blood tests and insulin shots. I sighed with relief and felt as if another small part of my normal life was being restored to me. I started to get to know my new team at Sharp Health in San

Diego. Dr. Brian had gone to Harvard Medical School and authored many books on heart transplant. He and his team followed me for about three years post-transplant.

While Dr. Brian was technically proficient, I felt like a bit of an outsider since he had not done my transplant. I noticed that he had lengthy conversations with those he had transplanted, while he barely spoke to me during my appointments. Missing a personal connection, I decided to return to Dr. Tom at Scripps to handle my post-transplant care. Dr. Brian and Dr. Tom actually know each other well and refer patients to each other on a regular basis. I prioritized my personal connection with my medical providers in making my decision to return to Scripps for follow-on care. I often encourage patients I visit to go with the team and hospital in which you feel the most comfortable. For me, this was Dr. Tom and Scripps Health.

As I mentioned previously, there is a bit of a "freak show" atmosphere when you are a recovering transplant patient and return home after the surgery. Thanks to Mary Shelley, one of my favorite authors, people are often fascinated with organ replacement and want to see living proof that it really does work. To quote Jimmy Buffet in his song "Schoolboy Heart," "Frankenstein . . . has nothing on this body of mine." I had many early visitors gape open-mouthed at my scar, which became a medal of valor for me.

Pat and I had been very low-key about my illness in our community. We are both private people and did not want anyone but our closest circle of family and friends dropping by for visits in the early days of my recovery. I encourage transplant patients to be selective about who they decide to see once they are home recovering. This is not elitism or rude behavior. Your body is tired from the surgery. Visits, no matter how pleasant, require effort and are often exhausting for the patient.

The week we returned home from Los Angeles, ten invited

visitors stopped by to offer their well wishes. In the following weeks, another thirty uninvited visitors came. When they arrived at our home, Pat played bodyguard, diverting many of them at the front door. If you are a recovering transplant patient, you must have someone posted as a sentry to help fend off unplanned visitors. You are not a circus side show; you are a person who has fought the battle for your life and need time to rest and recuperate. Those people, if curious enough, will find another way to contact you.

The other aspect to consider with uninvited visitors is germs. You will be wearing a mask for the first year post-transplant, except when you are alone in your home. With an immune-suppressed system, you must do this. I did not know that five years later masks would become ubiquitous as the world responded to a pandemic. I found fashionable masks with military-grade filter screens through a company called Vogmask. These high-grade masks kept bacteria and viruses at bay, which is a top concern as a transplant patient. Even a simple cold can put the mightiest of transplant warriors back in the hospital.

Of all the circus visitors, uninvited family members were the hardest. We soon discovered that some of our family members could cause us angst during these visits. Here is a true story of what happened to one of my fellow transplant patients. Several of her family members dropped by her home within a week of hospital discharge with two sick toddlers and an unbathed dog, all of whom raced into her living room unannounced. She did not have a gatekeeper to protect her from these people, and their germs could have made her very sick. She called me in distress from her bathroom and I drove over to her house immediately. I promptly kicked them out of the house and told them they could not visit until they were well.

They do not speak to me to this day, but my friend is alive and has learned to set limits regarding visitors.

Another suggestion is to have a "visitors' station" set up in your entryway. Pat and I had lots of medical supplies left over from my many hospitalizations. We had a large container of antibacterial gel, masks, gloves, and other items so that visitors could prepare to visit with me without bringing their germs. It was a small effort that kept my new donor heart healthy throughout the first critical year of recovery.

One final note: Family members or friends who annoy you before transplant will continue to do so after transplant, with even more intensity. According to the *Journal of the American Medical Association*, your cognitive brain function is impaired by some of the aspects of cardio-thoracic surgery. This can be temporary or forever, depending upon how much your brain was impacted during anesthesia. You can lose short-term memory. Your ability to cope with difficult people also decreases. If you are a cardiac patient who is waiting to get transplanted or has undergone surgery, go easy on yourself. Do not try to please everyone and focus on your recovery instead.

Let go of your expectations of yourself and others and embrace gratitude for getting a second chance at life. Your body and mind will heal faster, and you will feel more like yourself again.

The next lesson I learned as a transplant patient is that post-transplant, no one is allowed to jeopardize your health. Even people who say they love you and are family. They can wait. Maybe they can visit the real circus instead of creating one.

26

THE FIRST YEAR AFTER TRANSPLANT — A NEW NORMAL AND "HEARTVERSARY"

WITH A BACKGROUND IN BEHAVIORAL SCIENCE, I thought I was intellectually prepared for the first year post-transplant. In reality, my educational background did not matter one bit. Consider this: Until transplant occurs, you are surrounded by a literal army of medical professionals, social workers, psychologists and psychiatrists, and any other support needed to get you prepared for the surgery. Everyone is focused on one goal: To get the patient successfully through transplant.

After the operation and recovery, your medical team shrinks to your primary transplant follow-on doctor and a nurse practitioner. After being the focus of attention for a long period of time, you are left to ponder your "new normal" by yourself. Most likely, your caregiver has returned to his or her job to support the family, and you are now home alone or with your children and/or pets. You are left with your reconstructed body and the need to recreate your life. This is a lot harder than it sounds. There are limits on what the newly transplanted body can do. The patient must honor these limits and recreate his or her life to live with them. Many patients experience very high levels of fatigue that keep them from returning to work. Others go back to work within a few months. It is all an individual process.

I was transplanted at the age of fifty-one. I had worked full time with my cardiomyopathy condition until the age of forty-nine, when I was admitted for my emergency LVAD surgery. I had spent the last twenty-five years as a mom, wife, and working professional. Suddenly, my professional work role was gone. My two adult daughters had begun college and their careers and were making it on their own. The serious questions began to rattle around like marbles in my head: How was I going to rebuild my life? Who would believe that I could work again without the risk of serious illness? There was no guide-book or resource to answer these questions. I never felt so alone in my life.

Then I had a personal "aha" moment when I figured out that my life could be reinvented if *I made the effort.*

One morning, I grew sick of lamenting my isolation and decided to get busy. I was tired of being "the sick person" and decided to trade that role for a better one. I reached out to former colleagues and let them know that I was available for part-time consulting work in higher education. Two of them responded, and within a month I began working on small jobs to keep my brain busy. This helped me tremendously. I was coming up on my one year "heartversary" and it gave me a sense of purpose and meaning to be engaged professionally again.

While the professional work helped to offset some of our bills, it did not completely satisfy me. I felt so much gratitude just to be alive that I wanted to give back to my community. At Dr. Tom's request, I began visiting other LVAD and cardiac patients.

Things were going great with these patient visits until one

of them died while I was in his hospital room. It sent me into a tailspin of survivor guilt and worry. After this episode, I decided that there were many other volunteer opportunities available that would not cause me this type of anxiety. My good friend, Jim, the other transplant survivor who had visited me in the hospital, encouraged me to volunteer with him by leading a cardiac support group at Scripps.

Groups such as Mended Hearts exist so that patients can reach out and support other patients through their illnesses. Personally, these groups have helped me to get out of my head by helping others in need. They have taken me out of my house and put me back into the community. Jim and I have discovered through our volunteer work that two of the biggest problems facing transplant patients are *isolation* and *irrelevancy*. The isolation comes from having to give up former social and/or professional roles such as full-time employment, sports, or other activities. The irrelevancy comes from the isolation — feeling that you are no longer important to your community or job. I quickly learned that acts of service helped me to leave my feelings of isolation behind. For this reason, once you are through your transplant and feeling well, it is important to do what you can, where you can, to help others.

I encourage other patients to begin this process by leveraging their talents. For example, when I do not feel up to visiting people, I knit hats and scarves for them in red, which is the color symbolizing heart disease and recovery. Knitting is meditative for me and extremely calming. As I knit, I think positive thoughts for the person who will receive the item I am knitting. This is my small way of sending some TLC to another heart patient in the hospital. When I take the items with me on visits, people's faces light up as I put the red hat or scarf on them. The hospital is a very sterile, un-cozy place. The knitted items are my way of offering a bit of love and support to other patients. There are several knitting leagues in most areas for this purpose.

Here are some other examples of how transplant patients are contributing to their local communities. One transplant survivor, a female former chef, delivers heart-healthy meals to patients and their families free of charge for one month when they return from the hospital. This is an incredible act of service when patients and their families do not have the time or energy to cook. Another former concert pianist who had a transplant travels to hospitals all over Southern California to play soothing music.

The bottom line is, *giving back works*. It alleviates depression and makes the newly transplanted patients feel like they are a part of the community again. I started volunteering within my first year after transplant when my doctors gave me medical approval to do so. Please note: A transplanted volunteer must be cleared by his or her medical team before re-entering any public facility due to germs and bacteria.

Before I knew it, my first year "heartversary" arrived. I was happy, excited, and grateful. I had not experienced any rejection of my donated heart since the transplant. My husband and I decided to celebrate with a party for his birthday and my heartversary. We hosted brunch, read my donor family's letter, offered a long moment of silence to Alex in appreciation, and shared some of the highs and lows of going through the first year. It had been a crazy ride. We gave our friends and loved ones the opportunity to share or write in a guest book, offering their experiences along the journey with us. It was a fun and meaningful milestone in the long road to recovery.

It is critical to celebrate the events of your recovery. These milestones can provide you with positive insights when things get challenging in the years ahead. It is important to remember that transplant is *a treatment* for chronic heart failure, *not a cure.* Many people have remarked, "Well, you are right as rain now. You do not have to worry about any more heart illness." I wish that were the truth. I have known other transplant patients who have dealt with serious difficulties post-transplant, including infection and rejection. There is also the looming possibility that the donor heart will stop functioning and another transplant may be required. One of my friends was transplanted as a child and has endured three more transplants since his first one.

Instead of giving in to anxiety, I try to focus on my gratitude for each day rather than waiting for the next medical crisis. As most of my transplant friends say, "We are given the gift of time and extra innings."

The next lesson I learned as a transplant patient is that transplantation is a treatment, not a cure.

27

HEART TRANSPLANT RECOVERY: THE EARLY YEARS — 1-4

MANY PATIENTS I visit ask me if there is a "typical" heart transplant recovery process. The answer is no. Each person deals with so many factors: his or her anatomy, the quality of the implanted new heart organ, blood type, history of family illness, etc. There is an inside joke amongst CHF patients that "you pay your dues at one time or another." Some people struggle with years of cardiac illness prior to transplant, while others have a stand-alone incident such as a heart attack and are listed quickly. Many transplanted patients I know have had little to no complications following surgery, while others have required more surgeries, including additional transplants.

In my case, I paid my dues before my transplant. I died twice waiting for my new heart and was resuscitated by my medical and surgical teams. I was shocked by my AICD defibrillator over thirty times, but who is counting? I spent sixty days in a medically-induced coma on the brink of death. My organs had failed at a 95-percent level. Many doctors gave up on my chances of survival.

This turned around after my transplant. My body and organs recuperated quickly. I could breathe normally again and made a full recovery within six days. At fifty-one, my body was still young enough to come back from the brink of death. Every patient is different when it comes to post-transplant recovery.

Unfortunately, some patients continue to pay their dues after transplant. A close friend who had been waiting for a transplant for almost a year in the hospital was on a drug called Amiodarone to keep his arrhythmias away. We were helping him and his wife to cope with the process of waiting for transplant. We had encouraged him to list at Cedars-Sinai to increase his odds. He had already had an open heart surgery, and his chances of receiving a heart were not looking good.

After waiting in another hospital in San Diego for ten months, the medical transplant team finally found a good organ for our friend. We grew excited as he approached transplant.

Unfortunately, the Amiodarone pumped into his system during this time had left some negative side effects. After a successful twelve-hour surgery, his body went into acidosis and rejected the organ. He passed away within twenty-four hours of getting his new heart.

The program where this man was listed did ten to twelve transplants per year. At larger facilities such as Cedars-Sinai and the Mayo Clinic, the medical staff perform over two hundred transplants per year.

The transplant patient needs to be informed and realize that the choice of a hospital will influence the odds of receiving a suitable organ for transplant. It is a numbers game. Some patients have relocated from California to states such as Georgia or Alabama, since the number of donated organs available in those states is higher. This choice must be made carefully with thoughtful attention in mind, including the patient's insurance coverage.

Some patients also pay the price in terms of side effects from transplant. One of my support group members suffered a stroke after transplant and now has a condition called "drop foot." He drags his right foot when he walks, which has been very upsetting for him. Another friend was recently diagnosed with prostate cancer, which he believes he contracted due to the immune-suppressant drugs. These patients will probably never know if these conditions have been caused by their transplants, but they are left dealing with them, both physically and emotionally.

There is also the possibility of facing multiple transplants. One transplant friend had a serious heart condition since she was four years old. As she grew older, she needed to be re-transplanted three times due to her changing anatomy. Re-transplant is a distinct possibility for all of us, and a damn good motivator for making sure you follow your team's directives regarding your health and medications. Each person has to follow their own road to recovery and to do whatever is needed to maximize their opportunity for a healthy life post-transplant.

Ironically, most heart transplant patients do not die of heart disease. They die from other causes, such as cancer triggered by the immune-suppressant drugs. At the beginning of my fourth year out, I had four cysts found on my thyroid gland. This is a fairly common thing for women in their fifties. After a biopsy, they were determined to be benign. It was a scary process, but I stayed on top of it and worked through it. If they had been malignant, treatment to remove the cancer would have been available. I share with patients that the key is awareness, getting the medical information and data available through tests, and then acting accordingly. Information is power when dealing with a long-term chronic condition. While it is not always fun, it is necessary for survival.

The next lesson I learned as a transplant patient is that even the most successful transplants can result in immune-suppres-sant illnesses, such as cancer. Following the advice of your medical team is critical to long-term patient success.

28

DANCING WITH THE SCARS

FAST FORWARD TO JULY 2022. It is my first time competing in the Transplant Games of America as a transplant recipient. The only other competitors are those who are living organ donors, who compete separately. I am getting ready to enter the ballroom dance competition with my professional coach David Fan, who has spent two years teaching me the Latin-style rhumba and cha-cha dances so that I can contend for a medal. Alex's heart is beating wildly in my chest as we approach the dance floor. This is it. After two years of learning choreography and hoping for a medal, I walk hand in hand with David onto the dance floor.

My rounds go quickly, and the judges evaluate all the contestants, stony-faced. The event takes about four hours with all the divisions and age categories. I perform well but have no idea if I have medaled. I review my two routines in my head and am convinced that I have had a few missteps. Finally, the awards are given out by the judges. I am awarded a gold medal for my dancing in my age category. I am elated. I have met my long-term goal that I share with my coach, David, and I notice my family cheering me on as they place the gold medal around my neck. This medal is symbolic of my road to recovery, with all its detours and challenges. It now sits in a frame in my home office.

I am almost eight years out of transplant now as I finish this book. My body is strong and well, and I have returned to both work and exercise. I celebrate my gratitude by helping others to cope with the road to transplant and their recovery afterwards. I have created a "new normal" for myself consisting of dancing, training, walks, writing, consulting, lots of volunteering, some hobbies, and of course, fun. Advocating for women's heart health has become one of my new life passions.

If you are a patient who is facing transplant, I hope that my story has inspired you. I authored this book to help you and others by sharing my journey. While transplantation is a long road, there are many great medical professionals who will help you navigate your way. Transplant patients are warriors and survivors who are ready and able to help those who go down this road. At the end of this journey, we will all have scars. I hope you dance with your scars, too.

My final life lesson as a transplant patient features the work of Mother Theresa. She was quoted as saying, "Nothing makes you happier than when you really reach out in mercy to someone who is badly hurt." Even on my best day, I cannot begin to compare myself to Mother Theresa. What I can do is to place that phone call to a patient, visit someone who is waiting for their new heart, run a support group, or lead a transplant tribe. I challenge all other transplant patients to do the same. I will see you in our tribe.

EPILOGUE

AS I FINISH the edits to this book, it has been almost eight years since my heart transplant. I have been very fortunate in terms of my recovery. I have not experienced any rejection of Alex's heart. My overall health is very good. The only souvenirs I have from my transplant surgery are my scar and a small hernia that is golf-ball sized in the middle of my chest. My team tells me that this type of hernia is very common, and we don't need to worry about it. I try to live each day in gratitude for this amazing gift that was given to me.

My daughters are both healthy and have shown no signs of congestive heart failure. We did some genetic testing just to make sure they had all the care they needed. I am now down to a small dose of six pills that I take daily to keep my body from rejecting my new heart. I will be on these medications for the rest of my life. I go to my follow on team twice a year for check-ups. Our biggest concerns are infections and cancer, so I do the rounds with my dentist, dermatologist, general practitioner, and other medical teams to make sure I am in the clear. My days as a former sun goddess are now a thing of the past, as transplant patients are highly susceptible to skin cancer due to their immune suppression.

Pat and I have taken advantage of my good health and done a lot of traveling. People will often ask me if I am afraid to travel with my transplanted body, to which I respond, "Heck, no." I believe that God has given me extra innings to live this life to the fullest. And I intend to do just that.

Perhaps the hardest part for me was the decision about work-life balance. I used to be a workaholic, and my body paid the price. Now, I do contract work as a PhD consultant. I take the work when it comes. And try not to stress when it doesn't. I am still practicing at that. I am fifty-nine years old now, so I may do this for another five years or so, then dedicate myself to enjoying my life.

I think of Alex every morning when I wake up. I also like to offer small tributes to him in special moments. For example, last summer Pat and I walked up the Spanish Steps in Italy. Considering I could not walk five feet before my transplant, this was a major event for me. There are over two hundred steep steps that lead to a small but stunning chapel on the top of the hill. I felt Alex's spirit with me in every step and heard his healthy heart beating soundly. I entered the chapel and lit a candle for him. Then I wept. I am not one to cry in public, so this overwhelmed me. I looked up toward the altar, trying to hide my tears, and saw a beautiful sacred heart hanging above it. At that moment, I realized that God and Alex would always be with me on my transplant journey. It also occurred to me that I had really never been alone, even during the toughest parts of my transplant journey.

Some people have asked me if I carry any of Alex's "traits" with me. While there is a technical name for this in medical journals called "donor cell memory," I have not really experi-enced much of it. Some recipients report having new dietary challenges such as disliking a food they have always loved. I think this could be attributed to all of the changes one's body goes through with multiple larger surgeries. For me, I have noticed changes in a positive way, such as valuing every day as a transplant survivor and trying to live with less stress.

I wish you love, joy, and health on your travels, too. I have attached a resource page to provide assistance with the organizations I have mentioned in this book. I have included my own email if you would like to contact me. Thank you for reading my story. If I help even one other patient, I have accomplished my goal in writing this book and sharing it with you.

READER RESOURCES

WomenHeart Advocacy Group
https://www.womenheart.org
Email: mail@womenheart.org
712 H Street, NE Ste. 2201, Washington, DC 20002
Phone: (202) 728-7199

Thriving with Heart Disease: The Leading Authority on the Emotional Effects of Heart Disease Tells You and Your Family How to Heal and Reclaim Your Lives, by Wayne M. Sotile, PhD. Also see his website: https://www.sotile.com

Scripps Health Care System, Inc., La Jolla California
Dr. James T. Heywood, Clinical Director, Congestive Heart Failure Recovery Group
10666 N. Torrey Pines Road, La Jolla, CA 92037
Phone: (858) 554-5588

Author Contact: Darla A. Calvet, PhD
drdarlacalvet@gmail.com

ACKNOWLEDGMENTS

This book has truly been a labor of love with all of those who helped me. I wish to thank my editor Molly B. Lewis for the outstanding job she did on fine-tuning my story. I also want to acknowledge my publishing coordinator Leslie Ferguson for sharing her wisdom and guidance with me to make my final version of the book the best it could be. I am grateful to Acorn Publishing LLC for taking a chance on me and my story to help other patients. Thank you all.

ABOUT THE AUTHOR

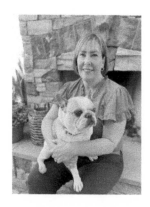

A heart transplant survivor, Dr. Darla Calvet won a gold medal for ballroom dance in the 2022 Transplant Games of America. Currently, she serves as the vice president of the board of directors for the Southern California Transplant Games of America team. She is also the CEO of Blue Tiger, Inc., a strategic planning consultancy. A doctor of education, Calvet holds degrees from Claremont Graduate University, San Diego State University, and the University of California at Berkeley. She lives in San Diego, California, with her husband Pat and their French bulldog Quinn, and she is the proud mom of two adult daughters, Claire and Annie.

Milton Keynes UK
Ingram Content Group UK Ltd.
UKHW012147041223
433798UK00012B/384/J